Chic & Slim
TOUJOURS 2

MORE
AGING
BEAUTIFULLY
LIKE THOSE
CHIC
FRENCH
WOMEN

Anne Barone

THE ANNE BARONE COMPANY

Chic & Slim Toujours 2:
More Aging Beautifully Like Those Chic French Women
Anne Barone

A Chic & Slim Book
Published by The Anne Barone Company, Texas 76309 USA

ISBN: 978-1-937066-23-9
Printed in the United States of America

Book and Cover Design: Anne Barone
Chic Woman Image Copyright © iStockphoto/ Yordanka Poleganova
Eiffel Tower Design: Joyce Wells GriggsArt

This book is intended as philosophy and general reference only. It is not to be used as a substitute for medical advice or treatment. Every individual's problems with the aging process are unique and complex. You should consult your physician for guidance on any medical cond-ition or health-issue and to make certain any product or treatment you use are right and safe for you.

For more links and related information visit:
http://www.annebarone.com

Contents

Dedicated to

All Those

Chic French Women

Who Age

So Beautifully

I am NOT my grandmother's 73 — and neither are you. Isn't that fantastique!

WHATEVER YOUR CERTAIN AGE, you likely look and feel more youthful than your grandmother did at an equivalent age. Older women are just not as "old" as they used to be.

True, the grandmothers of most of us went through difficult times— wars, depressions, financial difficulties, health problems—from which a good many of us have been spared. Additionally we have benefited from better understanding of nutrition and exercise, better medicine, more comfortable homes, more effective cosmetic products and procedures. Most of us are working, or have worked to earn an income, so we could buy the products and services to be healthier and more attractive.

Best, we have information. Much of that information is techniques used by chic French women who age so gloriously.

Many of you used the information in the first edition of my *Chic & Slim Toujours: aging beautifully like those chic French women* with spectacular results. But life in France and elsewhere has changed since that book was published in 2011. New lifestyle challenges generated new products and procedures to meet those challenges.

A totally new book was necessary to give you this new information and keep you aging beautifully. *Toujours.* Forever.

be chic, stay slim *toujours* — Anne Barone

Femmes d'un Certain Âge

THE FRENCH, known for *politesse* and diplomacy, do not say an older woman, nor a middle-aged woman, nor specify a woman's decade, they say a woman is *"une femme d'un certain âge."* A woman of a certain age.

The woman of certain—or uncertain—age is one who is no longer young, but without knowing her real age, you would have difficulty guessing it. She has taken such excellent care of herself and has such wonderful charm and chic, she may be older than she looks, but her real age does not matter. That is the sort of certain age that concerns us in this book.

The first edition of *Chic & Slim Toujours* (2011) analyzed a number healthy, active and chic women with ages from 43 to 99, an age span of 56 years. Sadly some of those women are no longer with us. We have lost the incomparable French actress Jeanne Moreau and the irrepressible YSL style muse Loulou de la Falaise among them.

In this new book you will find women you know well. You will meet others perhaps not so familiar who also give us role models for ageless, timeless beauty for which chic French women are so well known.

About the Author Anne Barone

ONCE FAT AND FRUMPY, in her mid-20s Anne Barone began to learn chic French women's techniques for eating well and staying slim and for dressing chic on a small budget. She lost 55 pounds and acquired a chic French wardrobe.

Chicer and slimmer, Anne Barone returned to the USA to find a nation growing sloppier and fatter. She decided to share her French secrets. In 1997, Anne Barone published her first French-inspired book *Chic & Slim: how those chic French women eat all that rich food and still stay slim*. More *Chic & Slim* books followed. This latest book *Chic & Slim Toujours 2: more aging beautifully like those chic French women* reveals the latest French secrets for dressing chic and staying slim in a woman's middle and later years.

Now 73, Anne Barone lives in Texas where she is attempting to create a bit of French Provence on the North Texas plains. "Far enough in the country to grow eggplant, garlic and lavender. But close enough to Dallas to make the sales at Neiman Marcus."

You can learn more about Anne Barone and *Chic & Slim* at the companion website *annebarone.com*.

Chic & Slim Books by Anne Barone

Print and eBook

CHIC & SLIM:

How Those Chic French Women
Eat All That Rich Food And Still Stay Slim

CHIC & SLIM ENCORE:

More About How French Women Dress Chic Stay Slim
—and How You Can Too!

CHIC & SLIM TECHNIQUES:

10 Techniques To Make You Chic & Slim
à la française

CHIC & SLIM TOUJOURS:

Aging Beautifully Like Those Chic French Women

CHIC & SLIM TOUJOURS 2:

More Aging Beautifully Like Those Chic French Women

CHIC & SLIM CONNOISSEUR:

Using Quality To Be Chic Slim Safe & Rich

ARMOIRE BOUDOIR CUISINE & SAVVY:

Success Techniques For Wardrobe Relaxation
Food & Smart Thinking

Using Toujours 2 for Success

SO MUCH IN FRANCE has changed since publication of the first edition of *Chic & Slim Toujours*. A new political party elected a new, youngest-ever French president. With him came a new French *Première dame*, who at 64 with her well-defined personal style, quickly became the new French icon of certain age chic.

In many ways Brigitte Macon's personal style and lifestyle are traditional. In other ways, she is creating new rules. In this new book we first look at Brigitte Macron to analyze how she exemplifies traditional French certain age style, then, how she is showing women a new, more flexible way of living and dressing in our current challenging times.

The second part of the book, is devoted to products and techniques that today keep certain age women looking beautiful and youthful. These are your how-to.

As the first edition of *Chic & Slim Toujours*, this new book is designed so that you may approach it as you would a menu in a French bistro. Not everything on the menu will be to your taste, that is, your personal style and lifestyle. But there is much useful information here. No matter your age, career, income level, ethnic background or personal style, you will surely find something delicious and satisfying.

Remember that chic French women's best anti-aging success secret is that they start early. I did. You should too.

A sense of freedom
is something that, happily,
comes with age and life experience.

Diane Keaton, *American Actress*

Brigitte Chic

BRIGITTE MACRON. She is French, chic, slim, and certain age. Since coming to our attention with her husband's announcement of his candidacy for French president, this now *Première dame* has become an object of fascination and extensive media coverage. Particularly for her personal style. She is the new chic French certain age style icon.

The French magazine *Gala* calls Brigitte Macron "the ambassadress of chic *à la française*" and says she dazzles by her ultra sculpted silhouette and her sense of style.

Nathalie Rozborski, trends specialist and general manager of the French image consulting firm NellyRodi told *Le Parisien* "Brigitte looks like the women we regard with pride."

Stylist Isabel Spearman, *The Telegraph* fashion columnist and image consultant in the UK declares Brigitte Macron "an icon of ageless style."

Of that style the French magazine *Le Point* wrote: "Sober, elegant, up-to-date and with just the right amount of audacity, the new first lady's wardrobe brings to the fore the excellence of French savoir-faire."

Gala adds more accolades calling Brigitte Macron *la reine du style avec une allure moderne et classe*. The queen of style with a modern and classy allure. *Une première dame qui ne manque jamais d'élégance*. A first lady who never lacks elegance.

As for her role as ambassadress of chic French fashion, Brigitte Macron told *France Info*: "When I travel, people talk to me constantly about the way I dress, of the importance of fashion, and I hear without cease that Paris is the first. We show the entire world we know how to dress, and fashion is totally part of our culture. It's an art, a total art, and I am very proud if I can contribute a little to give a form of visibility. It is very important for me."

Few French women have captured such world-wide attention since another Brigitte: Bardot in the 1950s—and she for the clothes she did not wear, more than for those she did.

Few other first ladies have set the fashion world awhirl since Jacqueline Kennedy came to our attention in the early 1960s as the wife of American president John Kennedy. A strong part of Jackie's allure was her youth: age 31—and that she was a number of years younger than her husband. A strong part of Brigitte Macron's allure is her age: 64—and that she is 24 years older than her husband.

Shortly after the French election, in her profile of the new French first lady in French *Elle*, editorial director Erin Doherty declared Brigitte Macron *"une femme exceptionnelle."* A romantic, like a heroine in a Françoise Sagan novel, courteous and bourgeois, living a passion made free by her exceptional choice. In the case of Brigitte Macron, her exception choice (at age 53) to divorce her husband of more than 30 years and marry a man who was not even born at the time of her first marriage. Tradition combined with modernity, says *Elle*.

In examining Brigitte Macron's lifestyle and personal style, what elements are long-followed French traditional practice? What are non-traditional and unique to her? While her husband Emmanuel Macron is working to bring about a "transformation" in France that will solve the country's serious economic and political problems, what transformation is Brigitte Macron bringing for a new, modern definition of chic French certain age style and lifestyle?

CHIC FRENCH STYLE TRADITIONS

First, let's look at the traditions of chic French style that form the basis of Brigitte Macron's personal style.

French women generally have defined their personal style by the time they are in their 30s. As years pass, they refine and update this style in response to changes in their lifestyle—and in their maturing bodies. The French women's magazine *Femme Actuelle* acquired and posted photos of Brigitte Macron dating back to the mid-1990s at *Lycée la Providence* in Amiens when she was teacher and Emmanuel Macron was then a student. The magazine has also posted a video clip from the couple's 2007 wedding.

The basics of Brigitte Macron's present personal style are evident in those images. The dresses with skirts well above the knee to showcase her shapely legs, the mid-length bouffant, very blond hair worn with bangs, her radiant smile lighting her face, and her bright eyes. The white dress she wore for her wedding to Emmanuel Macron in 2007 is very similar to the white Vuitton mod dress in which she was photographed welcoming American first lady Melania Trump to the Bastille Day 2017 festivities. She wore both dresses with very high-heels.

In one photo from the 1990s, this one a head and shoulders photo of Brigitte Macron, she bears a striking resemblance to Jane Fonda, circa the time the American actress won her Best Actress award for the 1971 film *Klute*. Jane Fonda was 34 in 1971. In 1995 Brigitte Macron was 42, we might note in passing. In those 1990s photos Brigitte Macron looks younger than age (then late 30s, early 40s) as she looks younger than her mid-60s today.

Brigitte Macron's certain age personal style is a refined version of what has long been her style choices. She admits to always having an interest in fashion and in being well-dressed. She told French *Elle*: "I am very enthusiastic about fashion. There exists a certain idea of the French woman in the world. I have always paid attention to how I dress. Ask my daughters or my students! I never go out of my house without being carefully dressed and my hair styled. It has been more or less successful. But I do not know how to do otherwise."

Chic French certain age women favor clothing in solid neutral colors. We most often see Brigitte in black or navy with some royal blues — and of course, the skinny blue denim jeans. Red appears from time to time in a blazer or top. She wore a bright red Vuitton dress with zip accents when photographed working at her desk in the Élysée Palace. A rare wearing of a print was the black dress with all-over white design she wore when the Macrons hosted Donald and Melania Trump at the Eiffel Tower restaurant in July 2017. Up to the time of this writing, Brigitte Macron's outfits have been usually in solid colors.

Chic French women traditionally wear the best quality they can afford. Though in more recent times pressure from the difficult economy and the influence of style icons such as Inès de La Fressange who regularly adds budget items in her daily outfits, have led chic French women to include lower-priced pieces. Good design is now available in budget versions—though this was not true in the past.

Since Brigitte Macron came into the spotlight when her husband announced his candidacy for the French presidency in November 2016, we have most often seen her wearing designer fashion. Most often thus far Louis Vuitton. Not surprising since, as reported by the French magazine Le Point, she has been guided in refining her personal style by Delphine Arnault, the assistant general manager of Louis Vuitton. Delphine Arnault is also the daughter of Bernard Arnault, chairman and CEO of Louis Vuitton, world's largest luxury-goods company.

Though usually to famous actresses, not politician's wives—for promotional purposes, Louis Vuitton does lend their fashions. Items are registered and checked out to the borrower, then checked in on return. Like the system used at your local library. Only in Brigitte Macron's case it would be a 2600 euro wool jacket, not the latest bestselling novel.

Brigitte Macron has also worn designs by French haute couture fashion designer Alexandre Vauthier known for the "sexy attitude" of his clothes. He has designed for Beyoncé and Madonna. In cold weather we see Brigitte Macron wearing her bright blue Moncler puffer jacket with jeans or black pants, and usually, her v-necked black tee shirt.

In shoes, she has a preference for Italian designer Gianvito Rossi's very feminine and sensual stilettos. She made headlines in the fashion media in November 2017 when she appeared on the steps of the Élysée to join her husband in welcoming Saad Hariri, the Lebanese prime minister. On this occasion Brigitte Macron wore a Louis Vuitton burgundy parma dress with burgundy Roger Vivier pumps. For ultra casual she has worn black New Balance sneakers.

Another point about Brigitte's shoe preferences. Most often we have seen Brigitte Macron wearing ultra high heels with pointed toes, a style that makes legs look longer and leaner. Most often her shoes have closed toes. A good choice for certain age, because at that stage of life toes are often not as pretty as they once were.

On the Macrons trip to Italy in summer of 2017, Brigitte did wear open-toed sandals, but the platform espadrille covered most of her foot. The burgundy leather of the sandals was a different shade of red than the bright tomato red top she wore. An example of how French women like to combine different shades of the same color in their outfit. Yet the two reds were separated by her skinny white jeans so their difference was not glaringly obvious. Toenail polish matched the burgundy leather of the sandals.

Brigitte Macron, we are assured by various media reports, does buy some of the fashions she wears. Of course, designs by top French designers are expensive. Thus coats and dresses in a neutral color are a long-term fashion investment that can be updated year to year with accessories in a trendy color. The fashion media were excited mid-November 2017 when for the ceremony for the victims of the Paris attacks Brigitte Macron updated her double-breasted with silver buttons black coat with a thick cobalt blue scarf around the neck and matching cobalt blue gloves.

Vogue US was one of several fashion media that posted an announcement and comments of scarf and gloves update. Titled *Brigitte Macron Elevates Her Winter Wardrobe With One Easy Piece*, the magazine wrote: "Macron wrapped up in a chunky, cobalt scarf that provided contrast and warmth with coordinating gloves. The leather gloves amped up the modern polish of Macron's directional look, mixing old world elegance and modern flourish. Macron's exposed zip booties provided a sleek finish."

We had seen the black coat, leather pants and boots last year. The cobalt scarf and gloves were new.

A traditional tenet of French chic is that a woman outfits herself in a manner that draws attention to her best feature or features. And often by directing the focus of a viewers gaze away from a less attractive feature. For Brigitte Macron, her legs are that notably best feature. Her dresses, even for formal evening wear, are always well above the knee. If the occasion or temperature demands pants, they are always formfitting skinny jeans or trousers. The only exception she has made thus far is when visiting the Shaikh Zayed Grand Mosque during the visit to open the new Louvre Abu Dhabi. To visit the mosque, she wore a white tuxedo trouser suit and covered her head with a long gray and white patterned silk scarf and walked barefoot through the mosque as religious protocol required. Modesty done chic.

While Brigitte showcases her attractive legs, she observes the tenet of keeping a less attractive feature covered. Rarely do you see her décolleté, that area on the upper chest just below the neck. This area can be a problem in certain age. Necklines are usually high on her dresses and tops. The one notable exception seems to be a v-necked black top that bares a triangle of her upper chest. The black top showed up under a bright blue half-unzipped puffer jacket while she was campaigning with her husband at a Pyrenees ski resort, and under a bright red blazer walking across the Élysée Palace grounds in the summer of 2017 and again under a beige blazer at the G20 summit a few days later.

Brigitte Macron follows the usual chic French certain age dictum of no plunging necklines nor pushup bras. Though she does have a generous bust. Unusually generous for French woman of her age and bone structure. That said, absolutely no analysis of Brigitte's physique I have read has made any suggestion of breast augmentation. Chic French women generally put out much effort on both leg and breast maintenance keeping these features optimum. Cold baths to maintain tone, for one thing. And there are many spas and beauty institutes in France offering leg and breast beauty treatments.

If chic French women wear eye makeup, they generally will forgo lipstick, at least any lipstick other than the palest shade. Likewise, if they wear color on their lips, such as that bright French red lipstick, they will skip the eye makeup. This is not a certain age tenet, but one generally followed by all chic French women, teens onward.

No matter whether dressed in jeans and casual top or the most formal outfit, Brigitte invariably has eye makeup, but only the palest color on her lips. Not only do the pale lips work well with her skin tone, but for someone who must spend much time eating and drinking "in public," it avoids the necessity for touch-ups. Though lipstick technology has advanced sufficiently that touching up lipstick is not the frequent necessity it once was. Eye makeup paired with nude/pale lips also avoids the necessity of a variety of lipstick colors to harmonize with outfits of different colors. On the other hand, it must be acknowledged that with chic French women's tendency to wear monotone outfits in neutral shades, that bright red French lip color looks good with them all. These women have figured all the angles, haven't they?

Traditionally French chic called for no color, only clear or pearl color on the fingernails. And colored, often bright red, polish on toenails of those beautifully pedicured chic French feet. In more recent times we see colored polish on the nails of chic French women, even chic French women of certain age. The actress Catherine Deneuve has almost always worn colored nail polish.

Today with the improvement in nail polish that is less damaging to nails and the health of those who apply the polish, we are seeing more color on fingernails of chic French women. Some are even wearing (gasp) nail art. Though almost all these women are young, not certain age.

Another way that Brigitte Macron is traditional: she uses personal style to communicate about herself. Shortly after Emmanuel Macron announced his candidacy for French president, Brigitte gave an interview to *Paris Match*. It was considered such a disaster that her husband felt the necessity of making a public statement explaining that his wife had not done well because she had no experience giving media interviews. Though I have read through that *Paris Match* interview several times and I fail to see the disaster. No doubt the disaster had to do with the nuances of French presidential politics at that particular moment.

In any case, for the rest of the campaign, Brigitte Macron principally communicated with the French people—and an enthralled international audience—through her personal style.

As I explained in the original *Chic & Slim*, for French women their personal style is as if they are wearing a signboard to tell people who they are and what they are about. An example of Brigitte Macron sending a specific personal style message was the outfit she wore to cast her ballot in the final round of the French presidential election. In *The Guardian*, Jess Cartner-Morley analyzed the message of the sleek Louis Vuitton navy coat, with a "face-flattering flash of silver leather in the raised biker-styled collar" Brigitte wore with leather pants:

> First, the biker-style collar made it a subtly rebellious look where, traditionally, political wives choose for election day

dutiful, church-on-Sunday coats or dull, senior-management-meeting ensembles. Second, Macron has worn this coat many times before, including—with leather trousers, that time—to Paris fashion week in March last year, so the choice emphasises Macron's own taste (this is from her wardrobe, not by order of an image consultant) and industry connections. Third, the coat is by Louis Vuitton, France's biggest luxury brand, and reinforces her husband's message of a progressive administration comfortable with big business.

STAYING SLIM TRADITIONALLY

Everyone agrees that Brigitte Macron has *une ligne parfaite*, a perfect figure. And her method for staying slim is a traditional one. We know one of the chief ways chic French women stay slim is by moderate amounts of good real food. While the *Michelin* starred restaurants serve up that legendary French haute cuisine, that is for special occasions. Chic French women maintain their slim figures eating plenty of vegetables and fruits served up in that plain cuisine *bonne maman* or French country cooking.

Recently Guillaume Gomez, chef *cuisinier* at the Élysée Palace, gave an interview to *The Telegraph* (UK) which revealed that in the traditional manner Brigitte Macron stays slim with good basic French cooking, meals that include plenty of fresh vegetables and fruits—10 different vegetables and fruits in meals every day. A healthy practice that surely Brigitte Macron's cardiologist daughter approves. A moderate amount of those good French wines and cheeses are also included.

Guillaume Gomez explained: "We serve only French products at the president's table if possible. Naturally the coffee isn't French, but all our fish, meat and fruit and vegetables either come from mainland France or from overseas territories. We prioritise local food produced less than 100 km from Paris for fruit and vegetables and some dairy products." Additionally the chef said that about half of the ingredients for foods prepared in the Élysée kitchen were organic. Some of the herbs, including rosemary and *laurier* (bay) are grown in the palace gardens. There are plans for an organic presidential vegetable garden on the grounds of either the Élysée or Versailles Palace.

In a televised interview the Élysée chef also revealed that helping in the Macrons' effort to eat healthily, he paid attention to using fruits and vegetables that were in season. He aimed for using the maximum variety possible. Of course, we know fruits and vegetables in season are at their peak taste. Variety makes eating healthy food more pleasurable and fights the temptation for between meal snacks.

When Brigitte Macron entertained children at the Élysée Palace to celebrate the Day of the Rights of Children, she introduced the palace chef and had Guillaume Gomez explain the work he does there. And explain that the chef's general guidelines are *dix fruits et légumes par jour et pas de junk food*. Ten different fruits and vegetables incorporated into the dishes served at the Élysée tables. And no junk food. The first lady assured the children, *"On mange très bien et on ne prend pas un gramme."* We eat very well and do not gain a gram.

Chic French women traditionally do not snack. Brigitte Macron's attitude toward snacking was made plain in a campaign documentary shown by the French TF1 and reported in *Paris Match*. Coming off the stage after one of the presidential debates, her husband the candidate feeling exhausted asked if any of the campaign staff had any "little chocolates or things like that." Brigitte cut in immediately: *"Non, je ne veux pas que tu manges des saloperies, tu vas dîner correctement."* No. I do not want you to eat rubbish. You will dine correctly.

Another chic French practice here. No exceptions to the no snacking rule. Even if you are exhausted, you do not give yourself a junk food boost. You eat good real food at meals.

But while President and Madame are eating well at the Élysée (at the expense of the state) the Macron administration knows that if the French citizenry are to eat a healthy diet rich in fresh fruits and vegetables, there must be some changes so that ordinary people can afford to buy produce. Unfortunately, as the French Agricultural Mutual Assistance Association reported, as of the autumn 2017 a third of French farmers have an income of less than 350 euros ($403) a month. That is only a third of the net minimum wage. Sadly one realizes the farmers might be making more money flipping burgers at a French MacDonald's.

In lieu of a wider food bill to help farmers hoped for the coming year, the Macron administration has brought about a signing of a "charter of commitment" between retailers and farmers. According to a *Reuters* report in November 2017, the main French retailers Carrefour, Casino, Auchan and Leclerc have signed this charter with French farm cooperatives, food producer groups, farm unions and industry representatives that will help ensure that farmers are paid a fair price for their produce. The aim is to allow them to earn a decent living while providing the country with healthy food.

Exercise, the other element in Brigitte Macron staying slim and healthy is also traditional. As of this writing I have not found Brigitte Macron quoted on the subject of her exercise. But we have seen the photos of her and her husband biking around town in *Le Touquet*, where they maintain a home. Various exercise experts have been interviewed by the media offering their guesses as to how Brigitte Macron maintains that perfect figure—and those marvelous legs—in her mid-60s.

In *The Telegraph* (UK), Peter Mac, one of top personal trainers in the UK for an A-list of clients, surmised that her slender frame suggested a lot of yoga, power walking, and low intensity body sessions. "I imagine she wants workouts that will keep her slender and toned."

Though Brigitte Macron's legs are exceptional, when she is photographed wearing sleeveless dresses, you can see that her arms appear to be those of someone in their 60s. These are not the sort of toned upper arms we became accustomed to see on the former American first lady Michelle Obama.

For more factual evidence of Brigitte Macron's exercise routine, the French news magazine *Le Point* reported that in August 2017 while the Macrons were vacationing:

> In the house on the Normandy coast owned by the lawyer Jean-Michel Darrois and his wife, photographer Bettina Rheims, Sunday mornings are lazy. While these tired Parisians slumber, Brigitte Macron does stretching and weight training exercises. An hour of gymnastics on the ground, for lack of a session of exercise bike. When the guests with crumpled faces arrive at breakfast, Brigitte Macron is waiting for them, impeccable and coiffed. Whatever her schedule was the day before or the duration of her night, Brigitte Macron gets up to exercise.

Here also is in operation what I call the French "always technique." Just as you always do not snack between meals, you always go through your exercise routine no matter how tired you are, or how little sleep you had the night before. And keep in mind that just because she is in her mid-60s, she has not abandoned her exercise routine. No doubt her cardiologist daughter also approves of this habit.

Medical research has demonstrated again and again that the best thing you can do to maintain brain and body is exercise. The best anti-aging technique is exercise.

FAMILY TRADITIONS
Traditionally, family is deeply important to the French. The home, or vacation home, of the grandparents, or great-grandparents, is often the regular rendezvous point for three and four generations.

For Brigitte Macron, family is deeply important. Both she and her husband have spoken about how the blessings of her three children by her first marriage was essential for their marriage. With their stepfather, Brigitte Macron's children and stepchildren form what *Gala* magazine described as *un clan très soudé,* a close-knit clan.

Her children's acceptance of their stepfather was aptly demonstrated by their support and participation in his presidential campaign. Particularly that of Tiphaine Auzière, the youngest of the three, who organized a campaign office for *En marche!* of the Opal Coast in Saint-Josse. She told *La Voix du Nord*, a regional newspaper in *Lille*, that she established the office on her own initiative because of the "faith she places in this man."

A charming photo on Europe 1 shows the pretty blond 32-year-old lawyer on a street corner with political leaflets in one hand and a food platter in the other, luring passersby to Macron campaign literature with thick slices of brioche.

In the more than a decade since the marriage of Brigitte and Emmanuel Macron, the rendezvous point for them with their children and grandchildren has been the Villa Monéjan that Brigitte Macron inherited from her mother. The villa built in the 1920s is located in the fashionable seaside resort town of *Le Touquet*, officially *Le-Touquet-Paris-Plage*. This small city on the northern coast of France is a holiday resort long popular with French entertainment celebrities and rich Parisians drawn to its long beach of fine sand, its tennis and equestrian centers, its kitesurfing and golf, its restaurants and shops, its nearby forest, and its luxury hotels such as the Hôtel Westminster, the elegant Art Deco style hotel built in 1924. Brigitte and Emmanuel Macron held their wedding reception in this hotel following their 2007 wedding in the office of the mayor in *Le Touquet's* town hall.

The town also has many well-preserved examples of the seaside architecture of the 1920s and 1930s. The principal designer of this architecture was Louis Quételart, one of the best known designers of seaside villas of this era. The style Quételart featured vast roofs, double gables and arches. Brigitte Macron's Villa Monéjan does not number among Quételart's villa designs, but in his villas you can see some inspiration from the Alpine style in which Monéjan and its neighbors in the "golden triangle," the most affluent area of *Le Touquet*, were created.

Tiphaine Auzière told *L'Express* that since her mother and stepfather married, the Villa Monéjan had become the family sanctuary, adding, "I also have beautiful memories of childhood here."

This spacious house of beautiful family memories that first belonged to Brigitte Macron's parents, what do we know of it? In June 2016 when Emmanuel Macron was being spoken of as a possible presidential candidate and the media and Internet were buzzing in reaction to the French taxing authority's upping the evaluation of the property, *La Voix du Nord* set out to investigate. The newspaper reported that this house in the coveted heart of the city with the nearby shops and amenities is a house of four stories built in the 1920s. The article's author, journalist Olivier Merlin, was able to talk with several of the Macrons' friends who were familiar with interior of the house. A 350,000 euros restoration done in recent years has brought the interior of this almost century-old house to an ultra-comfortable contemporary modern design—with a beautiful modernized kitchen. In back is a walled garden of several hundred square meters. One Macron friend was quoted as saying, "It's a fairly simple home in the end. Not at all a museum. A livable house."

No one has explained why those affluent families who built their seaside villas here on the English Channel coast of France in the 1920s chose an Alpine style of architecture. Ornate Swiss chalets with lots of gables and little balconies. (The area around the Macrons' villa is still today called by many Swiss Village.) When you look at one of the many photos of the Macron's villa that have appeared recently in the media, you cannot help but notice the exterior colors. The predominant colors are two shades of brown, a rich dark chocolate and a lighter milk chocolate, very much the colors of the Trogneux chocolates whose profits made the purchase of this family vacation home possible. Accent areas are the color of the candy's luscious creme fillings. Bands of red circling the building here and there suggest the bright red seen on lettering on the gold wrappers of the Trogneux *Macaron d'Amiens* and with which bags of these pastries them are tied. The villa's exterior colors appear an architectural tribute to the family artistry of Jean Trogneux Chocolatier for 5 Générations .

L'Express featured an article *Le nid douillet d'Emmanuel et Brigitte Macron au Touquet*, The cozy nest of Emmanuel and Brigitte Macron in *Le Touquet*. The article pointed out that the villa sits at the edge of the busiest street in *Le Touquet*. "Parisians, accustomed to narrow spaces, find it [the villa] superb, with its three levels of living space and its city garden. The *Touquettois* consider it "normal" when comparing it with the other properties of the *"Forêt"*, *le vrai quartier chic*—the truly chic district. The magazine comments that in the recent restoration work the villa has been given "a stroke of gray." All the railings and banisters have been painted in a creamy weathered gray that plays well with the two chocolate shades and the white and red accents.

In her comments about the family's time at the villa, Brigitte's youngest daughter Tiphaine told *L'Express* that: "When she finds herself in *Le Touquet*, the recomposed family has its routine. As soon as they arrive on Friday, they share a late dinner at *Brasserie Les Sports*, the cafe on rue Saint-Jean. Walk in the dunes with children and dogs. Rendez-vous at the beach near the colorful door [of the beach cabin] that good resident Brigitte Macron rents by the year. The children play while the adults talk." We also learn that grandpapa Emmanuel Macron makes a point of carrying a book during these weekend family gatherings as an encouragement to his grandchildren to read.

In preparation for his announcement as a candidate, the Macrons did allow *Paris Match* in April 2016 to observe one their weekends *en famille* at the villa. Since his election as president, time and security considerations make these sorts of articles less possible. So *Madame Figaro* sent Bertrand Duguet to *Le Touquet* for *Un week-end au Touquet dans les pas du couple Macron*, A weekend at *Touquet* in the steps of the Macrons, to give readers an idea on the life of the presidential couple on their visits to the villa.

The writer began his visit as the Macrons are known to do with a leisurely stroll along the beach enjoying the sea air and keeping an eye out for kitesurfers and the seals that regularly can be seen in the water. Then it was time to check out the restaurants where the Macrons are known to eat: couscous at the Villa Nomade or more classic French cuisine at Ricochet where duck breast is roasted with lavender salt. Table No. 10 is the Macrons regular table at *Brasserie Les Sports* where the speciality is steak tartare and, in the guest book, the article writer is impressed to see the names of Serge Gainsbourg and Harrison Ford. For actual sports, there is the tennis center where Emmanuel Macron is known to play often.

Then its time to check out the covered market of *Les Halles* whose architecture combines dark beams amid Norman arches, and where everything from clothing to fish is sold among an enormous variety of local meats and produce. As for the *bonnes adresses de la Première dame,* the shops that the French first lady is known to patronize, there is Perard fishmonger on rue de Metz and the butcher shop of Nicolas Kinget, the fourth generation of Kingets to supply the good people of *Le Touquet* with veal, beef and lamb.

Little surprise that the Macrons have sold their Paris apartment and made the Villa Monéjan in *Le Touquet* their principal residence. In any case, when they are in Paris, at least for the next five years, they have as a pied-à-terre the Élysée Palace.

After the election, the new French first lady confirmed to *L'Express* through a spokesperson that being *Premier dame* of France would not change her role as grandmother of seven. "Brigitte Macron has the intention of continuing to take care of her grandchildren, to pick them up at school as far as her schedule will allow."

She also wanted to reassure the French that the functioning of Élysée Palace would not be interrupted by the frequent presence of her children and grandchildren. She told *Point de Vue* magazine: "The Élysée is a place of work and official receptions and it will keep this vocation. Our family life, with our children and our grandchildren, has found naturally its place, but the major part of the time, outside the palace."

Most likely the Villa Monéjan will continue to be that place for children and grandchildren outside the palace where most of family time will be spent. *Gala* reports that the first couple reserves two evenings a week, one for family time, and the other, time with each other.

One reason the French believe time with family is so important is because it is then that children are educated in *l'art de vivre*, the French art of living well, so that life has pleasure and meaning. So that children learn the arts of eating and dressing and interacting with those with whom they live and work.

When *Elle* magazine asked Brigitte Macron about her own education, she responded that her schooling had been with the Sisters at *Sacré-Coeur d'Amiens* where "I did not look down, never. And I would not put into my head something I did not believe. I had a critical attitude very early on." She further explained that her valuable education had been from her family. "I was lucky to have incredible parents, and a very loving and close family. What they especially transmitted to me is respect for others. I could do everything, even bring back bad grades, but they were extremely strict about the respect we owed to each other."

An example of how this respect for others plays out in everyday life is an incident reported in *Le Courrier Picard*, a regional Picardy newspaper. In late November 2017 Brigitte Macron returned to her hometown of Amiens for an unannounced, non-official visit. The *Marché de Noël* was in progress and the spectacular Chroma, the sound and light show at the cathedral that is a highlight of the Amiens Christmas Market. Nicole, one of the longtime employees of the Trogneux family chocolate business, was working in the company's Christmas Market chalet.

And there is Nicole. Saleswoman for 36 years at Trogneux. So many years of friendship with Brigitte Macron. Nicole displays a radiant smile in the Trogneux chalet on place Gambetta. "I was busy and she appeared, smiling. It's always a great emotion [to see her]. She takes the time to pass. I knew her at the store when she was giving a helping hand. She has not forgotten anything of this while her life has completely changed," says Nicole, visibly touched. "I'm glad she finds time to enjoy her family and come to Amiens. She comes each year. But this is the first time as *Premier dame*. And her contact with people was done with naturalness," adds Nicole.

Brigitte's nephew Jean-Alexandre Trogneux who now runs the family chocolate business gives more insight into how the family influenced the children. This son of one of Brigitte's older brothers, and only eight years younger than Brigitte, in an interview with *L'Action Agricole Picarde* newspaper, spoke of Brigitte's father, his grandfather: "He was my best friend. He had an incredible openness, a great dignity and a rare ability to listen." Openness and a willingness to listen to the opinion of others and dignity are qualities people mention when speaking of the French first lady Brigitte Macron.

When nephew Jean-Alexandre speaks of how, under his grandfather's encouragement, he developed the passion he now feels for the artistry and marketing of his artisan chocolates and *macarons*, we find parallels to Brigitte's description of how she developed her passion for teaching: by working hard to gain the necessary skills, then doing the job as well as she possibly could. Always looking for ways to do the job better.

THE WORK TRADITION

Most adult women in France work. Of the developed countries in the world, France has the largest percentage of women in the workforce: 84 percent as of a recent tally. As *Slate* magazine summed it up in the title of their article "If America Is Hell for Working Women, France Might Just Be Heaven." In France, by the time the generous parental leave and stipends run out, the child is old enough for one of the excellent nursery schools. The French believe that the family is important and that giving parents institutional and financial support is a way to promote healthy and productive citizens.

Brigitte Macron married at 20. In the decade that followed, with her first husband, an international banker, she gave birth to three children: a son in 1975, now an engineer; a daughter in 1977, now a cardiologist; and another daughter in 1984, now a lawyer. In an interview given to the French magazine *Elle* several months into her husband's presidency, Brigitte Macron explained: "When my third child was born, I wanted to pursue another career. A friend told me that the Academy of Strasbourg, where we lived then, was looking for teachers, and as I had a master's degree in literature, I applied and was selected."

We English speakers who struggled through more advanced French classes with those near incomprehensible verb tenses and those pesky *conjonctives* and *circonstancielles*, may find comfort that, initially, when native French speaker who had been educated in a Catholic parochial school Brigitte Macron found herself teaching French grammar, she was equally confounded. She told *Elle*: "I had no idea. I had studied only literature! The first hour was dizzying. I spent fifteen days without sleeping, just working. And very quickly, teaching was a real happiness and even—maybe it's naïve—a pride. I never felt as good as coming out of a class that went well. When a class goes badly, however, it's terrible. Because we lost more than an hour, we lost the opportunity to transmit an author, a knowledge, a desire."

The family moved from Strasbourg to Amiens, the town where Brigitte Macron was born and grew up—and the location of her family's chocolate business. In Amiens, at the *Lycée La Providence*, she was teaching French and Latin literature and coaching the drama productions when she encountered a brilliant student who would later, in 2007, become her second husband. And who, ten years after their marriage, would become president of France.

As Chloé Friedmann wrote in *Madame Figaro*: "Even if 24 years separated lycée student and teacher, destiny would recapture them."

Whatever might have been the criticism and gossip about the relationship that developed between student and teacher, everyone agrees that Brigitte Trogneux Auzière Macron was a gifted teacher. She has a passion for French literature—especially the writing of Gustave Flaubert—that she passed on to her students. She told *Elle*, "Flaubert is the best tracker of stupidities of all literature. Everything in Flaubert is significant. My students did not have the right not to love him!"

For Brigitte, the genius in poetry is Rimbaud. And on her bedside table she says she keeps the work of another French poet, Charles Baudelaire's *Les Fleurs du Mal*.

Another first lady was a passionate admirer of Baudelaire. This one the American first lady Jacqueline Bouvier Kennedy, wife of American president John F. Kennedy. In 1951, in her essay for *Vogue* magazine's competition for its *Prix de Paris* (which she won), Jacqueline Bouvier, then a college student, in the required essay on people she would like to have met, one of the three Jackie named was the poet Baudelaire. She who had lived and traveled in France and studied at the Sorbonne in Paris was deeply knowledgeable of French literature and history. She had deep appreciation for French art and culture. For many of us, Jacqueline Kennedy was our "teacher" who conveyed to us her passion for France and its art and culture—and fashion—just as Brigitte Macron in her years of teaching passed on her passion for art and literature to her French students. And who is now passing on to the world her passion for French fashion.

For eight years after her marriage in 2007 to Emmanuel Macron, Brigitte Macron taught at *Lycée Saint Louis de Gonzague* in Paris. In the week following the election of Emmanuel Macron as president, *auFeminin*, the French women's publication, interviewed two of Brigitte Macron's former students at the *Lycée Louis de Gonzague*, often referred to as "the Franklin" for its location on the rue Franklin. The article featured the comments of Georges de Durfort who was in her French literature class and Nassim Helou who studied Latin. These former students described their teacher as "refined, fair, and well-educated." George de Durfort said that "*tous les élèves l'adoraient*" all the students adored her. He also described how at the end of each class, Brigitte Macron had a small ritual that consisted in picking at random a student's name so that student could recite orally what he had retained. "It was not a punishment, we even hoped to be chosen."

Nassim Helou commented that, unlike many teachers at elite schools such as *Saint Louis de Gonzague*, Mme Macron made a point of not differentiating good students from the lesser able ones. "She was a teacher who cared for and supported all her students."

Because her husband Emmanuel Macron had a position in the Hollande administration, Brigitte Macron was able to take her students to visit the Élysée Palace which houses the offices of the president and his staff. She also made possible for her students to meet Fabrice Luchini. (To help you place the French actor, Fabrice Luchini played the husband of the Catherine Deneuve character in *Potiche*.) A friend of the Macrons, the actor is also known for his theater performances reading French literature texts of La Fontaine, Céline, Baudelaire and Philippe Muray.

Shortly after Emmanuel Macron won the French presidency in May 2017, *Paris Match* interviewed Laurent Poupart. The director of *Lycée Saint Louis de Gonzague* the eight years Brigitte Macron taught there told the magazine: "BAM" [Brigitte Auzière Macron], as her students nicknamed her, was a professor in love with literature and, first of all, with her job, a real vocation. Her charisma, the strength of her words, her enthusiasm, transported her pupils. Joyful, optimistic, smiling, she was not stern but, thanks to a great natural authority, she commanded their respect."

When the magazine asked the director about how this wife of a high-ranking government figure fit in with the other teachers at the *lycée*,

Laurent Poupart assured them that Brigitte Macron's position did not change her behavior, nor that of the other teachers. Additionally, they had all benefited in that, through Brigitte, they had been able to meet France's new president before he was elected.

Brigitte Macron's first two careers: the first that of homemaker and mother, and her second that of teacher, prepared her for her third career, counselor to the presidential candidate. And prepared herself as a candidate for the role of France's *Première dame*. More than in previous French presidential elections, the personality of the presidential spouse was important to the French electorate who had unhappy memories of the melodrama involving the then President François Hollande's partner and his actress girl friend.

In campaign documentaries we see Brigitte Macron as her husband's speech coach, his nutritional guide, his opinion gatherer—and as *auFeminin* wrote: the candidate's *soutien omniprésent et infaillible*. The candidate's ever-present and unerring support.

The late financier and suburban shopping center magnate Henry Hermand, who was a longtime mentor to Emmanuel Macron and who died only weeks before his protégé's announcement as a candidate, knew the couple well. He was quoted by Richard Werly in *Le Temps*: "We forget too much that Brigitte is a teacher. She knows how to detect the potential of a young person, to cultivate it, to give them confidence."

Bernard Spitz, boss of the French Federation of Insurance and leader of the *Gracques*, the collective of intellectuals and technocrats who constitute the epicenter of the Macron universe said, "His success is not that of a couple. Macron alone is a Formula 1 of politics. But without a doubt she gives him that extra maturity that makes the difference."

According to one campaign staffer, Brigitte Macron also had the useful ability to read the eyes of journalists. An ability credited to her teaching experience. Remember the teachers who knew what mischief you were up to just by reading the expression in your eyes?

Summing up Brigitte Macron's value to her husband's presidential campaign David Chazan, *The Telegraph's* Paris correspondent, wrote:

> Her ability to shrug off setbacks and criticism while astutely assessing opportunities, has made her invaluable to her husband. Her toughness and drive, twinned with charm and a megawatt smile, played a fundamental part in propelling Macron, a relative political unknown, to victory against the odds in one of France's hardest-fought elections in recent memory.

> She drilled and coached him before make-or-break campaign speeches, re-assuming her early role as his drama teacher (a career she gave up to devote herself to her husband's political ambitions), carefully weighing and testing every phrase, and usually having the final say. Often acting as his harshest critic, she always coaxed him to do better.

David Chazan adds that her humor and "allure rock" style helped her fit in with the rest of the campaign staff who were mostly millennials.

Surely no one would ever downplay the value to candidate Macron of having continually at his side a wife who was *toujours très, très chic*. And a showcase for the best of French fashion. All three previous careers prepared Brigitte Macron for her fourth and current: that of France's *Première dame* and its ambassadress of chic French fashion.

During the campaign Emmanuel Macron had stated that, once elected, he would propose a statute to give the role of president's spouse an official status. Such a statute would provide a budget and a staff much like the system for presidential spouse in the USA. (In 1978 President Jimmy Carter signed a law that provides for a budget and a staff for the first spouse, a staff that in recent years has numbered between 16 and 25 people according to Rice University's Baker Institute.)

But the French people were much opposed to the idea of the statute. A petition against it quickly gained over 300,000 signatures. The first reason against the statute was that, under the current system, money covering the expenses of the *Premier dame's* activities and projects comes out of the Élysée budget. The statute would mean separate funding. The frugal French could not see the point of allocating additional funds. And Macron's political opponents did not want to give any sort of aid to this woman who was such an asset for the president.

The petition was not against Brigitte Macron, but against the position of a *Première dame*. Robert Schneider is an authority on the wives of French presidents. His book *Première Dames* was published in 2016. In an August 2017 article in *Le Figaro* titled *Depuis Valérie Trierweiler, le rôle de première dame est devenu impopulaire*, Since Valérie Trierweiler, the role of first lady has become unpopular, Robert Schneider explained:

> [French first ladies] have all been more or less popular, until the "drama" Trierweiler. The latter was the first very unpopular first lady. By her sometimes aggressive intrusion into the public debate (we remember her famous "tweet"), her role even less official because she was not married to the head of state, and her stormy history with the latter, she has permanently degraded the position. Since the five-year period of François Hollande and the grotesque episode of the scooter, a rampant hostility exists against the role of first lady.

Alix Bouilhaguet, a journalist who covered the spouses and partners of the 2017 presidential candidates was quoted saying. "The French first lady cannot be someone who whispers in the ears of the president. We had that with Valérie Trierweiler. She created a blurring of the lines, and people didn't like it."

So despite the petition, despite the abandonment of the idea of a statute to make the first lady position more official, Brigitte Macron is nevertheless France's *Première dame*. Plan B is an allocation of 440,000 euros per year out of the Élysée budget. A charter of transparency provides for a public accounting of Brigitte Macron's activities in her first lady capacity and the money spent for these activities.

In the *Elle* interview in August 2017 after the project of a statute had been abandoned, author Erin Doherty wrote:

She knows the importance of the so singular function that she occupies, the vagueness that surrounds her position, and that a charter of transparency should contribute to enlighten the sometimes excessive expectations and the criticisms so prompt to fall. Behind the blond hair that serves as a shell, she hides her doubts. And, as any good anxious person, she knows the only avenue: work. Every morning, in her office in the Élysée, she sets her daily schedule on sheets of paper, with a fountain pen.

Sheets of paper! A fountain pen! Surely those 440,000 euros will cover a smartphone appointment calendar app.

Erin Doherty continues:

Nothing predestined her to find herself in the Élysée. And yet, in a year of campaigning she became a symbol in the world, and in three months of First Lady, this impossible job, she found her right place. How? Because she is above all the wife of Emmanuel Macron and that, for him, she is ready to assume everything, or to fade away. Meet an exceptional woman, whatever she says

Exceptional woman. And, as 84 percent of French women, she works. Premier working woman of France.

TRADITIONAL, BUT NOT *AU COURANT*

First legs. Then hair. When Brigitte Macron first came to worldwide media and social media attention in late 2016 with the launch of her husband's presidential campaign, her most commented on feature was her very shapely legs. Her next most commented on feature was her hair. The ultra blond long bob definitely requiring a lot of upkeep was not the haircolor-hairstyle combination most chic French women were currently wearing. Certainly not most chic French women of certain age.

I place Brigitte Macron's hair between the traditional and non-traditional sections of this Brigitte commentary because, in some ways, her choice of hairstyle follows chic French tradition. In other ways, she is definitely breaking tradition. At least some current definition of how a chic French woman of certain age should wear her hair.

Brigitte Macron's haircut is one English speakers call a bob and the French call *le carré*, literally the square. The *carré* is a classic French hairstyle. Some of us remember this hairstyle worn by singers Mireille Mathieu and Juliette Greco—after Juliette trimmed the long, untamed locks that had been her signature style in the smoky cafés frequented by the existentialists early in her career. Also the French actress Mireille Darc, whose passing we noted recently, wore a bob very much the length and shade of blond we see now on Brigitte Macron. Women all over the world have worn it in one version or other since women began "bobbing," that is, cutting their hair in the early 1900s.

The French catalog numerous versions of *le carré*. Brigitte Macron's haircut is *le carré avec franges*, the bob with bangs. The magazine *Femme Actuelle* in their analysis of Brigitte Macron's hairstyle termed it *un carré blond platine*, a platinum blond bob and analyzed it as, "A very strong haircut that gives personality to her face."

In the first media reports commenting on Brigitte Macron's hair, the English language media often referred to her hair as "peroxided." The writers of these articles seemed to ignore that the hair of many women in their mid-60s does not require bleach to remove the natural pigment. Biology takes care of that. Though we do not know what part, if any, of Brigitte's blond is natural.

The French language media generally avoided *"peroxidée."* But *Elle* magazine did use the term *blondissime*, a reference to a product line of L'Oréal for rendering one's hair blond.

So what had so many people *bouleversé* about Brigitte Macron's hair? If you read French style publications lately, you have the definite impression that the greatest concern among French women today is not that there might be another of those horrendous terrorists attacks France has experienced in recent years. No, what worries chic French women most seems to be that someone might think that their hair appeared *trop travaillée*—that effort had been put forth in the color and styling of their hair—though, in fact, a large number of products and techniques are required to render that totally natural "undone" unworked look.

Then, into this milieu of the no obvious effort for hair mindset came Brigitte Macron, a chic, expensively-dressed certain age woman who appeared to have had definite work done to achieve the color and styling of her hair. Also, the currently acceptable natural look requires that hair not look dry nor show any sign of frizz. Brigitte Macron's hair showed evidence of both, especially in the early photos that we saw.

The ultimate test for a hairstyle of course is whether it suits the person: Is it right for their hair and shape of face, and their personal style? For a French *Première dame* Brigitte Macron's hairstyle seems to be working well. In an analysis of her hairstyle the magazine *Femme Actuelle* praised her haircut because it "softens the oval of her face. This long and slender, almost plunging, bob is ideal to soften a jaw that is a little too square. Her features appear younger and more awake." The magazine also thought the bangs did a good job of camouflaging her forehead wrinkles, yet still allowing some of the forehead to show through. And, as a sign that people were becoming more accepting of her blond haircolor, the magazine praised her haircolor as, "neither too golden nor too silver, and complimenting her skin tone."

Gala magazine called the haircolor "a very luminous and sexy color that suits her perfectly."

Le carré Brigitte does well for both casual and very dressy. For the inauguration of her husband as president in May 2017, with her powder blue Louis Vuitton suit she wore her hair in a classic French chignon, what the French call *chignon banane*—and what we in the USA in the 1960s called a French twist. When the Macrons welcomed the president of

Lebanon, to accompany the ultra sophisticated black dress by Lebanese designer Elie Saab, Brigitte's chignon was the *chignon bas de danseuse*, a bun worn at the base of the neck as many ballerina's wear.

By styling her hair in more traditional French hairstyles and picking a haircolor that suits her personal style rather than the trend of the moment, Brigitte Macron was defying the current pressure to look "undone." As I write this, however, in the most recent photos of Brigitte, I note that her hairstyle is evolving toward the unworked style. In a photo taken of Brigitte in a cafe sipping a mulled wine 28 November 2017 when she made a personal visit to the Christmas Market in her hometown of Amiens, her blond bob is noticeably longer on her shoulders than previously. Styling is more relaxed.

VARYING FROM THE TRADITIONAL

Now we come to those ways in which Brigitte Macron is different from the more traditional chic French women of certain age.

For Americans who endured decades of caustic comments and criticisms from our French acquaintances about our big smiles and our unnaturally white dentistry-assisted teeth, Brigitte Macron's megawatt smile and gleaming even teeth, major components of her successful personal style, give us definite satisfaction.

Those decades ago, I always noted that the models and personalities in French women's magazines, particularly those that catered to the French middle class, often had a crooked tooth—certainly not those perfect teeth we saw on the models and personalities in magazines published in the USA. Rarely were these French teeth brilliant white. The women did not often smile. Certainly in my real life chic French acquaintances, a bemused smile was the closest they came to hilarity.

In Harriet Welty Roquefort's writings about her life in France, this author of *French Toast* and other books, tells how her French stepsons are mortified when she laughs out loud. For chic French women, audible laughter was long considered *vulgaire*. Now we learn that Brigitte Macron laughs out loud.

Philippe Besson, author and friend of the Macrons, told *The Telegraph* of Brigitte Macron's self-deprecating humor. Self-deprecating anything is not a traditional chic French attribute. But attitudes are changing. Not just with Brigitte Macron. But self-deprecating humor is evident in some of the interviews that another French fashion icon Inès de la Fressange has given of late.

Brigitte Macron's often quoted comment about her husband: *"Le seul défaut d'Emmanuel, c'est d'être plus jeune que moi."* The only fault of Emmanuel is that he is younger than me, caused *Gala* magazine to call Brigitte Macron "the queen of the punchline" for her ability to respond to criticism with humor—often self-deprecating humor. She is also very adept at throwing out responses to tough questions with historical references: Jupiter, Jeanne d'Arc, Montaigne. And she is refreshingly frank, it is noted. Frankness is not always the case with political spouses who often choose circumvention.

In *Elle*, Erin Doherty writes of Brigitte Macron: "She is all that one says about her: spontaneous, laughing, sympathetic, empathic." For those of us who in decades past were acquainted and frequently socializing with chic French women, those four terms would not be the descriptive terms we would have chosen. More likely: reserved and calculating, serious, and totally uninterested in another woman—and certainly not interested in another woman's opinions or concerns.

But here we have Brigitte Macron, one of whose chief assets for her husband's presidential campaign was the ability to carry on conversations with strangers and learn their opinions and concerns.

Of course the most obvious way in which Brigitte Macron does not follow the traditional pattern of most chic French women is the relationship with her husband. Difficult to find in France—or anywhere—another couple whose relationship is exactly like that of

Brigitte and Emmanuel Macron. Especially in that she is 24 years her husband's senior. Their relationship is certainly unlike any of the recent French presidential couples.

The French newspaper *Le Monde* summarized: "For the first time in a long time, it is a bonded couple who will enter the Élysée. Before the sentimental vaudeville of the incumbent president, Nicolas Sarkozy, a few weeks after being elected, had been left by his then wife, Cécilia Ciganer. Jacques Chirac and his wife, Bernadette Chirac, each occupied a separate apartment at the Élysée. François and Danielle Mitterrand had not shared a daily life for a long time."

This summary leaves out (because it had been referred to in a previous paragraph) President Macron's immediate predecessor François Hollande leaving his partner Valerie Trierweiler abed, and, helmeted, speeding through the night on a scooter to an assignation with his actress girl friend.

After these preceding presidential couples, here come the Macrons happily married. Shock! Especially since marriage as an institution is definitely on the wane in France with couples opting for civil unions, or simply forming a family unit without any official sanction. In any case, French marriages have never been known for monogamy. They rarely involve the kind of closeness and seeming inseparability that the Macrons demonstrate. As *Le Monde* goes on to point out:

> Brigitte Macron, 64, will be a first lady in her own right as she was a totally involved candidate wife. Because it is together that this atypical couple has climbed the steps of power. Daily field trips, meetings, TV shows, meetings of *En Marche!* ... She took part in every moment of her husband's ascent. Not as a mere accompanier, stooge or *compagne pot de fleurs*, but a real actress in this battle.

No doubt Brigitte Macron is happy that this prestigious French newspaper does not consider her a "companion flower pot."

Another political publication, the French language *Le Temps* assures us that Brigitte Macon is not a *potiche*, a trophy wife. Richard Werly who interviewed Brigitte Macron early in the campaign wrote: "The other great asset of Madame Macron is to be everything except a *potiche*. Her knowledge of French and Latin literature, her natural taste for conversation, her ability to be simple when nothing is simple."

Brigitte Macron told the political columnist: "Write well that I am a normal woman. I do my shopping like everyone else. I'm not disconnected." She added, "Hiding me would not make sense. Nor would being on the front of the stage either. I am where I must be: at his side. Never far away."

Celebrating his victory in the first round of the voting, Emmanuel Macron told the audience., "*Toujours présente et encore davantage, sans laquelle je ne serais pas là.*" "Always present and even more, without whom I would not be here".

Philippe Besson traveled with the Macron presidential campaign and authored a book about Emmanuel Macron as candidate titled *Un personnage de roman*, Like a character in a novel. The writer explained the Macrons' relationship in an interview with *Paris Match* in September 2017: "He would not have won without her. She is inseparable from him."

Philippe Besson described the Macron relationship as "fusional," a descriptive term for a relationship where the two people are acting and needing to be as one person. He continues:

You have to remember where they come from. Brigitte Trogneux-Auzière is a girl from the provincial bourgeoisie who marries a man at 20 and has three children. Then, at 40, she meets a young man of 16 years. Together, they face hostility, misunderstanding, disgrace. Anyone who has been discriminated against collapses— or develops an unshakable determination. This is their case. On a daily basis, he needs her to be there. And she knows that he needs her, so she's there.

What does Brigitte Macron say about the relationship? Between the first and final rounds of the election, she told *Le Journal de Dimanche*: "Our functioning as a couple intrigues. Emmanuel and I, we believe that it is better with two. And since it's hard, we share. I think it's a lot nicer than being disjointed. I would have a hard time living differently."

By chance, shortly before the Brigitte and Emmanuel Macron came to my attention, I had been reading Sarah Bakewell's *At the Existentialist Cafe: Freedom, Being, and Apricot Cocktails*. The book focuses on the couple most closely associated in the public mind with existentialist philosophy, Jean Paul Sartre and Simone de Beauvoir. In their intellectual fusion, the Macrons remind me of the famous Existential couple. But with major differences.

Sartre and Beauvoir worked every day side by side discussing their work and following a commitment to "tell each other everything." Sarah Bakewell assures readers that the romantic aspects of the Sartre-Beauvoir relationship were disbanded in the early years and each went on to other lovers. A lot of other lovers. At the end of the work day, Simone de Beauvoir went home to her apartment, Sartre went home to his apartment—that he shared with his mother. Brigitte and Emmanuel Macron are together 24/7.

Brigitte Macron told Alix Bouilhaguet, author of *Le Couloir de Madame*, a book on spouses of the candidates in the 2017 French presidential election, "We do not know how to do one without the other."

THE BRIGITTE MYSTIQUE

Mystique. That ability to reveal enough about yourself that people will find you interesting and want to know more—without revealing so much—or something negative—that causes people to loose interest in you. Even avoid you.

Having considered the ways in which Brigitte Macron is very much in the tradition of chic French women of certain age—and the ways in which she differs—we will look at yet one more chic French tradition that she exemplifies. For Brigitte Macron, as for any woman with a well developed mystique, that mystique is, in its very nature, unique.

Chic French women are unusually adept at creating a mystique. At the moment of this writing, not yet one year into the presidency of her husband, Brigitte Macron has a stellar mystique. Both *l'amour* and *la mode* are important to the French. The Macrons with their unusual love story, and Brigitte's role as a new chic French style icon—not just certain age style, but French style in general—and her willingness to use her position in the media spotlight to promote French fashion has generated a desire to know more about this woman. Three years ago almost no one had heard of her. Three years ago she was teaching school, for heaven's sake. Now she is France's *Première dame*. And she has those extraordinary legs she shows off in haute couture—at age 64.

The Macrons have assistance managing their mystique. Early on in the campaign they put themselves in the hands of a professional. Mimi, that is Michèle Marchand, image consultant and head of Bestimage, one of the country's most powerful celebrity photo agencies. As a strategist for the Macron campaign, Mimi convinced the Macrons to reveal more about portions of their lives than is common with most French politicians. We likely would not know as much about their relationship but for the decision, that because the early student-teacher phase of their relationship was a potential political liability, it would be better to put the facts out—before other versions began to spread about what Brigitte Macron has described as "this senseless love."

So during the campaign we learned some facts. Still there is much we hope to know about what factors played a role in creating this unusual woman. Not from blatant curiosity, but in the hope we might use the information to improve our own lives and appearance. Just as in the early 1960s many of us wanted to know more about the American first lady Jacqueline Kennedy so that we could be more stylish and refined.

We have not yet seen in English a biography of Brigitte Macron such as Mary Van Rensselaer Thayer's 1961 book *Jacqueline Bouvier Kennedy* in which Mrs. Thayer called upon her knowledge gained as society columnist for newspapers in Boston, New York and Washington and her diplomatic contacts and world experience to give such an intimate portrait of the American first lady that, for years, people whispered that Jackie surely had written the book herself. In the book we saw delightful photos of the youthful Jackie and in the early years of her marriage, we learned about her years at Vassar and her life in Paris when she studied at the *Sorbonne*. Jackie Kennedy was only 31 in 1961 when she became America's first lady. Brigitte Macron was 64 when she took on that role for France, the age at which Jacqueline Kennedy Onassis died.

In the early 1960s, our information about the American first lady was limited to magazine and newspaper articles, infrequent television and personal appearances, and the book and imitators it inspired. Today with the Internet, if you read French, you can often find three or four new articles about Brigitte Macron each day. Even in English you might locate one or two. Brigitte Macron Wears Balmain for World AIDS Day in France. Brigitte Macron: the 5 reasons she is not on social media. Brigitte Macron, 64, steals the spotlight away from her husband in Senegal. *Brigitte Macron à la rencontre d'agricultrices en colère.*

Yet as much as we know about Brigitte Macron, this woman's mystique remains strong. Because the overriding question that can never be answered—because these things can never really be totally and truly analyzed—is: What was it about this woman on the eve of middle age, this teacher and married mother of three, that so attracted a teenage boy of great intelligence and promise that he decided that this woman—and only this woman—was necessary to his success and happiness in life?

Keep in mind, when Emmanuel Macron's parents became concerned about the relationship that had developed between the drama workshop coach and their teenage son, they did not ship him off to a sheep ranch in the outback of Australia. No, they made arrangements for him to attend an elite *lycée* in Paris. Paris! A city that has as many beautiful, intelligent, fascinating women per square kilometer as any city in the world. Surely one of those *Parisiennes* would have made him forget the high school teacher in Amiens. But, no. For Emmanuel, it was Brigitte and only Brigitte.

Then there is the other side of the question. What was it about this woman that lead her in her mid-50s to be persuaded to divorce her husband of more than three decades and marry a young man of 30 who, after earning several degrees was only beginning a career as a civil servant? And Brigitte was a woman accustomed to a comfortable life, first as the child of an affluent bourgeois family, then the wife of an international banker. In divorcing her husband and marrying this much younger man, she was, by any standards, taking a big gamble.

In a video released by the Macron campaign during Emmanuel Macron's presidential bid, there is a segment of the couple's wedding in *Le Touquet* in 2007. We see the couple taking their vows before the mayor. Then, there is Emmanuel making his speech at the wedding reception. He looks youthful, and his expression is that of the kid who has just won the most wonderful prize in the world.

For someone like me who had for weeks been viewing photos of the new French first lady with her megawatt smile, these video clips created something of a shock. Between the beaming groom and the camera sits Brigitte. She does not even look at her new husband as he speaks. She certainly is not smiling. In fact, I have never seen a less happy looking bride in any wedding video. Her decision to enter this union with this man could not have been without apprehension.

Yet, even if the mysterious dynamics of physical and emotional attraction are never completely knowable, we do have clues to the mystery of the Macrons' relationship. These clues lie in French literature and French history about which both husband and wife are knowledgeable and passionate. First let's look at French literature.

To someone well-versed in the jewels of 19th century French literature, the idea of a young man of ambition and promise in a relationship with an older woman who serves as a mentor who propels him on his way to success—and, in many cases, is his lover as well—is not unusual.

First, there is Balzac. *La Comédie Humaine*, the series of 19th century novels written by Honoré de Balzac is considered a realistic portrait of post-Napoleonic French life. Balzac's rich cast of characters contains a number of promising young men in relationships with older women.

In *Yeats the European* edited by A. Norman Jeffares we get a good summation of the young men and older women in Balzac's novels courtesy of the Irish poet W. B. Yeats. In 1905, Yeats bought a set—all 40 volumes—of Balzac translated into English. As Yeats read, surprisingly swiftly, through these many volumes, he noted:

> The situation of being in love with a woman some years older and of superior social station is one inhabited over and over again in the *Comédie*, and from every possible perspective, especially in the scenes of Parisian life. Raphael and Foedora, Madame de Beauséant and d'Ajuga-Pinto in *Le Père Goriot*, Rastignac and Delphine de Nucingen in the same work, Lucien de Rubempré and Madame de Bargeton, d'Arthez and La Princesse de Cadigan: — in Yeats' words, a "beautiful high-bred woman" is adored by and frequently severed from a younger man, usually of genius. 'It is only a woman's last love that can satisfy a man's first love.'

> The woman of superior status, more worldly but perhaps no less idealistic than her lover, or perhaps much less idealistic, being Balzac's repeated type.

Yeats may have particularly noticed Balzac's characters' tendency toward involvement with older women because Yeats himself preferred younger women. Much younger women. Particularly later in the poet's life. But by that time Yeats had no need, as Balzac's young heroes did, for a older woman mentor to launch and further his career—either in politics or in literature. Yeats had already served two terms as an Irish senator, and in 1923, won the Nobel Prize for Literature.

Then, in Stendhal's *The Red and the Black*, there is Julien Sorel. In Charles Van Doren's *The Joy of Reading: A Passionate Guide to 189 of the World's Best Authors*, the academic and literary critic describes Julien Sorel as a young man of "energy, imagination and courage—with brilliant eyes though which his genius shines." Julien Sorel is set on his "startling progress toward wealth and power" by the aid of Madame de Rênal, the older woman with whom he falls in love.

Van Doren, by the way, considers *The Red and the Black* one of the two best books written in French, the other Stendhal's *The Charterhouse of Parma*. Van Doren believes that reading this saga of Julien Sorel is "an overwhelming experience."

Writer Philippe Besson is a Macron family friend. In a *Paris Match* interview about his book *Emmanuel Macron: Un personnage de roman*, Emmanuel Macron: Like A Person in a Novel, he was asked what character in a novel Emmanuel Macron most resembled. Philippe Besson's first response was Julien Sorel of *The Red and the Black* because of "the romantic side, the epic, and also for the love of an older woman Mme de Rênal."

When the interviewer reminded Philippe Besson that Emmanuel Macron had described himself as Balzacian, the author agreed that he [Emmanuel] has a little of Balzac's character Rastignac, in that he is "young man who has gone to the capital, a banker and a liberal. But he does not have the cynicism of Balzac's hero." Still, Emmanuel Macron's cultural tastes are *historique* and *classique*, anchored in the past, not in the popular culture.

Brigitte Macron has a passion for Gustave Flaubert, author of *Madame Bovary*. Flaubert is also the author of *L'Éducation sentimentale*. This novel published 12 years after *Madame Bovary* is not as well known perhaps to English language readers (Henry James said that in comparison to

Madame Bovary, that *Sentimental Education* was "dead.") Still, this story of the young man Frédéric Moreau and his obsession with an older woman Madame Arnoux was one of the most influential novels of the 19th century. A sort of negative self help book. Frédéric Moreau's story is a demonstration of how a young man of great potential can make bad decisions and cause great difficulties in his life. The inherent lesson in his story is how, by making opposite decisions, intelligent and ambitious young men can become happy successes. Such as become Minister of the Economy at age 36, and president at age 39 perhaps.

French history also gives us examples of young men put on the road to success by the older women with whom they fell in love. The theories of Enlightenment philosopher Jean Jacques Rousseau laid a foundation for our political and educational systems that have carried over to our time. His ideas played a major role creating the ferment that resulted in the French Revolution. Rousseau's thinking might never had the great influence on our history had it not been for the guidance and financing he received from the wealthy noblewoman Madame de Warens that began when he was 15 and she 29. Rousseau always considered Madame de Warens "the greatest love of his life."

EMMANUEL & BRIGITTE & HENRI & DIANE

Of course the historical figures the Macrons' appearance in the public sphere immediately brought to many minds were the 16th century French king Henri II and his mistress and advisor Diane de Poitiers. The latter is such an important figure in the history of chic French certain age women that I wrote about Diane de Poitiers in the first edition of *Chic & Slim Toujours*. For that book, much of my information about this extraordinary woman of the French Renaissance and her relationship with King Henri II came from *The Serpent and the Moon: Two Rivals for the Love of a Renaissance King* by HRH Princess Michael of Kent. Princess Michael is a direct descendant of Diane de Poitiers—as well as of Catherine de Medici, Henri II's queen.

More recently we have another book *Queens and Mistresses of Renaissance France* published by Yale University Press. The book is written by Kathleen Wellman, Professor French, Intellectual, and Early Modern European History at SMU, Dallas. Both these books are sources for much, though not all, information on Henri II and Diane de Poitiers that I use in comparing them with Brigitte and Emmanuel Macron. For brevity I will distinguish between the two sources by identifying the material as either from "Kent" or from "Wellman."

To begin, we will acknowledge that Henri II was a hereditary king in the period of the French Renaissance—and Emmanuel Macon is an elected president of the French Republic in modern times. Yet both are French heads of state in the system in place at the time of their service. And, true, Diane de Poitiers was a royal mistress, not a wife, as is Brigitte Macron. But we must keep in mind that in the French Renaissance, wives of kings (or future kings) were chosen for political reasons: to seal alliances between countries or to bring in new territory in their dowries. Henri II's wife and queen Catherine de Medici brought in her dowry a good chunk of Italy—along with all those Italian recipes that would serve as the basis of French cuisine. A queen's most important function, however, was to provide male heirs for the king since France's Salic Law prohibited female rulers. Potential queens had to undergo extensive physical examinations to evaluate their likelihood of producing many healthy children.

But a mistress was different. Wellman writes: "A mistress was chosen for other purposes. A king singled her out for his own happiness, generally on the basis of a sexual attraction. The mistress, whom a king selected for sexual pleasure or love, buttressed his masculinity. Her beauty sanctioned his choice."

Of course a king might have several mistresses, but a royal mistress was the special one. A royal mistress could be defined as "the woman the king would have married if the system had been different." Thus, a royal mistress is a reasonable equivalent of a wife in modern times. And certainly Diane de Poitiers' relationship with Henri II was more that of a modern wife than most royal mistresses of the French Renaissance. As stated in the Kent book: "Diane de Poitiers was the choice of the king's heart. If he could have married her, he would gladly have done so."

One thing absolutely in common between Henri II and Emmanuel Macron is that they met their loves at an early age and their devotion did not wane. Wellman wrote of Henri II that "Henry was smitten at a young age and remained so." We know from hundreds of media articles that Emmanuel Macron met Brigitte when he was a *lycée* student and she a teacher. He was smitten at a young age and remains so.

What most called to mind the comparison between king and mistress and the president and first lady was the age difference. Diane was almost 19 years older than Henri. Brigitte Macron is 24 years older than her husband.

As for physique and brain power, the two heads of state differ greatly. Henri II was tall and handsome, a gifted athlete, but his early intellectual promise had been badly interrupted by his four years as a hostage in Spain from age seven to eleven. Afterward Henri was, everybody agreed, chiefly interested in physical not intellectual matters. Released from Spanish captivity and back in France, Henri was gauche and bad mannered. His father, the king, François I was so appalled by Henri's behavior in the court, that he early put Diane de Poitiers, then lady-in-waiting to his mother Louise de Savoie, in charge of improving his son.

Though of medium height and slim build, from the earliest age, Emmanuel Macron has been considered brilliant. A charmer, who excelled academically, especially in writing. He does not seem to have been much active in sports as a teenager, though we do know that today he takes tennis instruction. He has been photographed pedaling around *Le Touquet* on his *bicyclette*. Brigitte was also photographed bicycling. These bicycle rides through the crowded streets of *Le Touquet* at the height of the tourist season are surely the closest approximation to the frequent gallops on horseback through the forest, the form of exercise that Diane and Henri shared.

Both Diane and Brigitte initially played the role of teacher for their later loves. Not only did King François I put Diane in charge of improving Henri, but shortly after the king's wife Queen Claude died leaving her six living children motherless, Kent tells us: "The king turned to Diane and appointed her to care for the royal children, the greatest honor he had shown her to date." Of course, Diane did not physically take care of the children, there were literally hundreds of servants dedicated to their care. Jean II d'Humières, a cousin of Diane, was officially governor of the royal children. Jean d'Humières, and later, after his death, his wife, deserved the royal trust placed in their childcare expertise. They were parents of 18 children.

While we have, of course, no photographs of Diane de Poitiers, there exist numerous paintings and descriptions written by her contemporaries. And there is the tapestry. Once part of the decor of Anet, the Renaissance chateau that Henri II had built for Diane, *The Drowning of Britomaris* now hangs in The Metropolitan Museum of Art in New York City. Kent tells us, "Scholars generally agree that the figure of Diana in the tapestry is as true a portrait of Diane de Poitiers as exists."

If you enter *The Drowning of Britomaris* in an internet search box, it will give you the link to the page on The Met website where you can see a large colored image of the tapestry.

Wellman describes Diane: "tall and slender with very white skin, red-gold hair, and blue-green eyes." Kent adds to the description telling us "Diane had a long neck and muscled arms and legs from riding. She epitomized the image of her era's beauty." In fact, so extraordinary was Diane appearance, many in Renaissance France believed that she accomplished her beauty by witchcraft.

We, with the benefit of more scientific knowledge in the 21st century than people in the 16th, understand that Diane's beauty was original pleasing features whose best she brought out with careful diet, regular exercise, ample rest, and a sensible skin care routine. Kent writes:

> Summer and winter in all weathers, she would rise at dawn and bathe her whole body in ice-cold rain or well water. She breakfasted with a cup of bouillon before leaving at first light for a brisk three-hour ride through the woods and countryside around Anet. On her return she would rest, and around ten or eleven, she would eat a simple meal. Only then did Diane de Poitiers begin her public duties as the widow of the Grand Sénéchal, attending to the affairs and greeting the growing number of her callers. She would dine at six in the evening and retire to bed early.

We also know that Diane avoided the makeup of the day that ruined so many women's complexions—and sometimes poisoned them.

> Diane's only beauty aids were a powder made of musk and rosewater and a paste used against wrinkles that she mixed herself, from the juice of a melon, crushed young barley, and an egg yolk mixed with ambergris [a waxy, grayish substance formed in the intestine of sperm whales and found floating in the sea or washed ashore]. She applied the paste to her face like a mask. Whenever Diane was alone, she slept propped upright on deep pillows to avoid creasing her face.

Brantôme, the chronicler of his age, who visited Diane de Poitiers, tells us that in her 60s, she looked 30. For centuries chic French women have been following Diane's guidelines to remain attractive and youthful.

As for Brigitte Macron, since the beginning of her husband's presidential campaign we have seen many media photographs. Like Diane de Poitiers, Brigitte is slender, blue-eyed, youthful looking and blond, though her shade is platinum. She prefers a bronzed skin tone. Brigitte is not tall, only about 5 foot, 4 or 5 inches. Her long, shapely legs and very high-heeled shoes she wears give an impression that she is taller than she actually is.

Brigitte is not considered a ethereal beauty as Diane was. Her photos from earlier years show an attractive woman with spectacular legs, but she was not, as a previous first lady Carla Bruni Sarkozy, a top fashion model. Brigitte married at 20, was a mother and homemaker for a decade before becoming a school teacher. She fascinates now for her perfect figure maintained into her mid-60s and for the fashions she (with a little advice and help from Vuitton) adorns herself.

Other than the one article, previously mentioned, that suggested that Brigitte rises early for a regular workout, we do not know at this stage specifically her exercise routine. Nor do we have specifics on her skincare program. We do know from comments by the Élysée chef that she eats a sensible diet, free from junk food and rich in fresh vegetables and fruits. While no one has accused Brigitte Macron of maintaining her attractive, youthful appearance with witchcraft as they did Diane de Poitiers, there have been denigrating comments on social media about Botox and cosmetic surgery.

Much that has been written about both Diane de Poitiers and Brigitte Macron is untrue—or, at least, distorted. Not always easy to sort out truth from falsehood. When reading about either woman, it is necessary to consider the source of the statements, and any bias, either positive or negative, that source might have. For Diane de Poitiers, some of the most slanderous statements came from Protestants in retaliation for her support for their persecution during the French 16th century religious wars. Slander of Brigitte Macron often comes from her husband's political opponents. And from other women jealous because they do not have her dedication and discipline.

Both Diane and Brigitte had been previously married. Oddly we know more about Diane's husband Louis de Brézé who lived and died four centuries ago, and his life with Diane, than about Brigitte's former husband André-Louis Auzière and the Auzières' more than 30 years of marriage. M. Auzière was born in Cameroon where his father was a colonial official. M. Auzière was a banker. *C'est tout!* Diane and Louis were only married 17 years. Married at age 15, Diane was widowed at 31 when Louis de Brézé died at age 73. Louis was 39 years older than Diane.

Considering that Diane's husband was almost four decades her senior, perhaps it did not seem so unusual to her that there were less than two decades between her age and Henri's. When Henri became king, he was 28, Diane was 46. Brigitte Macron has pointed out that she was the youngest of six children, her oldest brother 20 years older than she. Big age differences seem normal to her. When Emmanuel Macron was inaugurated president, he was 39. Brigitte was 64.

For both couples the relationship can be described as a partnership in every area of their lives. Even though a citizens' petition halted Emmanuel Macron's attempt to give official status to his wife's first lady position, as political columnist David Chazan wrote in *The Telegraph*: "Not only is Brigitte the beloved wife of the President—she is also his closest political advisor." Of Emmanuel Macron's inauguration, *The New York Times* wrote that it was also "the advent of a new kind of first lady for the nation, and a new kind of political partnership."

Kent writes: "Diane de Poitiers did not assume the role of an official royal mistress. She saw herself as the king's partner—someone he could trust, love, and in whom he could confide. At court and in public, Henri always referred to Diane as "Ma Dame"—"My Lady," which signifies the true relationship between them. His subjects called her "Madame" just as they would a sister or daughter of the sovereign. She was his fair Lady in the true chivalric sense." In fact, the relationship was conducted with so much propriety and discretion, many believed the relationship between Diane and Henri to be platonic.

Both Diane and Brigitte are fashion icons of their time. Before she was widowed Kent tells us Diane wore green and white, most flattering to her red-gold hair and luminous white skin. After Louis de Brézé died, she wore black as a sign of perpetual mourning. This color accented with white was equally flattering to her hair and skin.

Kent described the black and white dress Diane wore to Henri II's coronation:

> Her habitual deep, wide décolleté, draped with pearls from one shoulder to the other, was of black velvet, setting off to perfection her white skin and fair coloring. Her long black velvet skirt opened in front to reveal a white satin panel covered in gold and silver embroidery. She wore great pear-drop pearls in her ears and her hair was as always *à l'escoffion*, in a snood [an ornamental hairnet worn over the hair at the back of a woman's head] of trellised black velvet ribbon studded with pearls. On the top of her forehead, she wore a diamond crescent as her crown.

Brigitte Macron frequently wears black or white, or combinations of the two. But she does not limit herself to those colors. (Though it must be noted that Diane adopted black as a sign of her widowhood.) Fashion Editor Bethan Holt wrote in *The Telegraph*: "For her husband Emmanuel Macron's Inauguration as French President [Brigitte Macron] opted for a powder blue dress and jacket by Louis Vuitton, which she accessorised with pale beige high heels and a neatly elegant top handle Capucines bag, also by Louis Vuitton." Brigitte's hair was not in a snood, but was done in an attractive, sophisticated chignon.

Both Diane and Brigitte were born into prominent and affluent families. Both had comfortable lifestyles in their first marriages.

Both Henri II and Emmanuel Macron were improved by their relationships with the women they loved. Kent writes:

> Diane became a member of [Henri's] Privy Council and largely controlled the others. In every appointment, observers could see her sure hand guiding the young king. Those who had openly opposed Diane in the past were amazed that, instead of taking her revenge, she gave them appointments if she felt that they could be of use to the kingdom. Without the help of brilliant men in the key positions of his government, Henri's reign would not have

been described by the Italian ambassadors as one of the most remarkable in French history for the wisdom of its policies. They wrote home with nothing but praise for Diane's wise counsel, and declared that, as a result, the king filled his time "only with things useful and honorable.

In Emmanuel Macron's recent meteoric rise we see Brigitte's "sure hand." Between his graduation from the elite *Lycée Henri-IV* in Paris and their marriage, according to his well-sourced resume on Wikipedia, Emmanuel twice failed his entry exam to the *École Normale Supérieure*. He earned a master's in philosophy then worked as an editorial assistant to the French Protestant philosopher Paul Ricoeur. Then back to study for another master's degree, this in public affairs at *Sciences Po*. After an internship in Nigeria, he held several French civil service jobs. Nothing remarkable.

Then in 2007 Emmanuel Macron and Brigitte married. By the next year, 2008, Emmanuel Macron is no longer a civil servant, he is a highly paid investment banker at *Banque Rothschild & Cie*. In 2012 he is Deputy Secretary General in the office of President François Hollande. In 2014 Minister of the Economy. In 2017 president of France—at age 39.

How much political influence Diane de Poitiers actually had in the reign of Henri II, is still being debated by historians all these centuries later. Though it is unlikely that she was "ruling France" instead of Henri, as some have suggested. Given that today France is a democracy, we can be certain that Brigitte Macron will not "rule" France during her husband's term in office. It will remain to future historians to evaluate what influence she exerted on the politics during her husband's presidency. And it will only be in the future that we will know if Brigitte Macron's mystique is as enduring as that of Diane de Poitiers who continues to interest and intrigue three and a half centuries after her death. In 2017, in France the *Grand Prix de la Biographie politique* for best political biography went to a new book on Diane de Poitiers.

Legs

THOSE GREAT FRENCH LEGS. Chic French women are known to maintain attractive, shapely legs even in certain age. Lately we have seen an excellent example of chic French certain age legs. With above the knee skirts and tight skinny pants as mainstays of her personal style, French first lady Brigitte Macron has given us many opportunities to view her spectacular legs. Her legs would be impressive at any age, but the fact that she is 64 makes them even more so.

What is Brigitte's Macron's secret to such great certain age legs? While I have no specific knowledge of what the French first lady does as leg care, I do know much about how French women in general get and keep their *ooh-la-la* legs. In the first edition of *Chic & Slim Toujours*, one of the longest sections was on legs. That information is still valid and useful. But in this book I have more for you.

Chic French women believe that good legs are essential to their beauty and health. As with skin care, they are always availing themselves of the latest techniques, products, devices and medical advice. Interesting to me that French women's magazine articles on leg beauty often include information on which, and what percentage of cost, these leg treatments are covered by the French national health insurance.

Additionally, chic French women know neat tricks for making their good legs look spectacular. Further along in this chapter we will look at those. And before we discuss techniques and products that create and maintain pretty legs à la française, it is useful to understand the underlying philosophy. Chic French leg philosophy distilled to its simplest: Poor circulation is the cause of problems—dimpled orange peel skin (cellulite) and spider and varicose veins— that make legs ugly. Heat is the enemy of pretty legs because heat causes poor circulation. Cool is the friend of pretty legs because cool aids good circulation. Applications of cool counteract heat and thus aid circulation. Pretty legs must be maintained by regular care. Legs benefit from professional tuneups done in a beauty institute or spa. Serious leg problems should seek medical treatment at first symptoms.

This philosophy has developed from traditional practices and solid medical evidence. So how does this philosophy work out in real life? What do you need to do to have chic French legs? First, stay slim. Excess fat which insulates has a negative effect on circulation. Then, take cold baths or showers. Hot baths are avoided because not only can they cause vein problems for the legs, but they can also make breasts sag.

Cold baths and showers have long been practiced by chic women from the 16th century royal mistress Diane de Poitiers who was said to look 30 at age 60, and including American actress Katherine Hepburn who followed the advice of her father, a medical doctor, who advocated cold baths for general health.

Katherine lived to 96 and always looked radiant.

Though medical research has found definite brain and body benefits from cold baths and showers—as defined by one in which the water temperature is below 70 degrees F. (21 C.) you should gradually accustom yourself to the practice. For certain health conditions you MUST gradually become accustomed to colder water. To do otherwise is dangerous. One technique as outlined in the Healthline Newsletter:

The ideal way to take a cold shower is to ease in to the habit. Start by slowly lowering the temperature at the end of a usual shower.

Get the water cold enough that you start to feel uncomfortable. Then, stay underneath the water for 2 or 3 minutes. Breathing deeply will help decrease your discomfort in your mind. The next time you try this exercise, make the water slightly colder. Try to last for another minute or two in the colder water. After performing this activity 7 to 10 times, you'll find that you might even look forward to turning the hot water down.

If this idea interests, you can do further research and find a adaptation method that you can tolerate. For those who want to limit the cold shower to the legs, there is the method outlined in the first edition of *Toujours* that I found described on the *auFeminin* website. To perform this technique you need one of those shower heads attached to a hose that can be handheld. Standing in the tub or shower, you hold the spray nozzle about four inches from the skin, and beginning at the big toe bring the spray upward to the inside of the knee, then descend on the outside of the leg down to the ankle. Repeat 20 times alternating legs.

I can handle this procedure in warm weather. But in cold weather it is difficult even in a warm bathroom. So you cannot imagine how happy I was to read in *Madame Figaro* the advice of Dr. Joëlle Cohen-Pognot, Paris specialist in vascular medicine, who described her version for treating the legs with a spray of cold water. "But be careful: do it by gradually lowering the temperature because the veins do not like cold shock. Direct the jet from the ankle to the knee in a circular motion. "

That gradual lowering of water temperature I can tolerate, even taking the stream of water up to the top of my thigh so that my entire leg has a circulation boost as some vascular specialists advise. But even with gradually cooling water, I still need a warm bathroom.

While most French women learn effective leg care from their mothers, grandmothers and aunts, French women's magazines regularly remind readers of tried and true practices and alert them to new products and treatments. Useful to look at what these articles advise.

The French *Elle* frequently features advice for beautiful legs. Articles often appear in a July issue. These are timed to prepare readers to show their legs at their best for that month of August vacation at the beach. Of course, the articles all focus on how to avoid that dreaded hot weather malady: *jambes lourdes*. Heavy Legs occur when as the result of elevated air temperatures the blood vessels in the legs dilate and become congested interrupting the natural contraction in the veins and making legs, especially the thighs, feel hot, and as if they weigh a ton.

In *Comment en finir avec les jambes lourdes?* How to avoid heavy legs, the magazine outlines a leg program for your holiday time at the beach. In the morning do a leg massage with one of the gels or lotions specifically aimed for preventing heavy legs. During the day, instead of lying in the sun, walk briskly along the beach. Let the cool sea water splash on your legs to revitalize them. Be sure to wear light colored clothing that does not restrict circulation. Eat plenty of fresh fruits and vegetables for their vitamins and antioxidants that tone and protect veins. To aid circulation, drink green tea and take Vitamin B3 especially if you have a tendency for water retention. In the evening before bed give yourself a foot bath in cold water, or end your shower by a jet of cold water on your legs, lower calves to the thighs. At night sleep with your legs elevated. If your legs feel hot and heavy, put towels soaked in cool water on your legs.

The article also includes information on technology to fight the heavy legs condition, specifically the Climsom mattress-topper. This is a mat through which temperature-controlled water circulates, warm or cool as you choose. The cool temperatures work to decongest legs by reducing redness, feelings of warmth, swelling and discomfort and thus improving circulation in the legs. The Climsom (about 400 eruos) is available across Europe and in the UK. In the USA, there are similar products. The ChiliPad Cube is pricey at $500 for the twin and $1000 for a king. The Cool Buddy (cool temperatures only) is more affordable at $150. On my side of the Atlantic, these devices seem most often used by women dealing with hot flashes that interrupt sleep and those who want to save on their summer cooling bills by setting the thermostat higher at night and using the pad for direct body cooling. The motors of all the models make a humming sound that disturb sleep of some.

For something a little less high tech, but in a variety of very chic designs, the *Elle* article suggests thong style sandals with an elevated toe. The *Sveltesse* by *Royal Thermes Institut* is designed to eliminate cellulite, firm skin and aid circulation in the legs. The sole elevated at the toe slopes upward eight degrees requires learning time to be able to walk in them without falling on your nose. To get results from these thongs (flip-flops) you need to walk in them three hours a day.

While I have never worn the *Sveltesse* thong sandals, I did, several years ago, purchase walking shoes with the same angled sole that promised to give a better workout than a normal walking shoe. I was not willing to spend the amount of time necessary to learn to walk in them. When I returned the shoes to the store, the saleswoman just smiled and said, "Everybody brings these back."

In a more recent French *Elle* article *Nos conseils pour affiner nos jambes en quatrième vitesse* Our advice to refine our legs in fourth gear, gives more advice on improving legs because they are "a key symbol of femininity." The magazine advises *l'aquabiking* and *le Pilates* for refining the legs. In the USA *l'aquabiking* is usually called aquacycling. Basically it involves riding an exercise bicycle that has been lowered into a swimming pool. Proponents claim that this water version of cycling offers a safer biking experience with even better benefits than regular cycling. *Shape* magazines quotes physical therapist Alice Holland: "Aquatic exercises help to strengthen while protecting from joint pain and reducing injury," Chic French women think it is an excellent way to tone legs and the cooling effect of the water will combat any conditions that might cause "heavy legs."

As for Pilates, it is one of the best ways to elongate and lengthen the body and give the appearance of being taller and leaner. Years ago one of the *Chic & Slim* readers gave me a Jennifer Kries Pilates toning and sculpting DVD . I wore out the disk I used it so regularly. When I learned that the DVD was no longer in production, I bought two used disks as insurance. No other workout suits me better and gives me better results. Many other good Pilates programs are available on DVD and you can surely find one that suits you well. You can find classes in many cities.

Twenty years ago when I wrote the original *Chic & Slim: how those chic French women eat all that rich food and still stay slim*, chic French women did not go in for vigorous exercise the way women did in the USA. You did not find it among the recommendations for slimming legs. But the chic French attitude toward vigorous exercise in the role of leg maintenance (and general health maintenance) is changing. I am continually being surprised. Reading the January 2016 French *Elle* I was startled to see an article that offered advice for how to slim your legs *rapidement*. In the past, chic French women were not so likely to look for the quick fixes. The article presented the advice of a *coach sportif* who advised: *Après un échauffement cardio de 20 minutes, faire sa séance de musculation en répétant bien les séries. Après cela, on file courir pendant une demi-heure.*

Had I read that correctly? After a 20-minute cardio warmup, do a session of weight training. Follow that with a half hour run.

Cardio warmup? Weight training? Run? I checked to make certain I was reading a French magazine.

However, embedded in this article was a more traditional style of leg toning, a video of an eight and one-half minute workout. While you would be unlikely to work up a sweat, it would surely improve your legs. And even if you did not understand the spoken instructions in French, the instructor was dressed in cute striped leggings and neon orange trainers. Having recently struggled to understand the moves of an exercise video I was working with because the camera angle made it difficult to see exactly what the instructor was doing with her arms, legs and feet. I was impressed with the cleverness of using clothing to make the information more comprehensible. Those neon shoes let you see where her feet were at all times.

Running may be fine for younger women. But by the time a woman is well into certain age, in choosing her exercise, she must evaluate the benefits from that type of exercise versus the possible injury it might inflict on aging muscles and joints.

Walking is a wonderful exercise that can be done without placing your body at risks other types of exercise would. Most health experts agree that a brisk 30 to 45 minute walk at least five days per week will give you a good certain age workout. Now that I am in my mid-70s, I follow the recommendation for three 10-minute walking sessions per day. This is advised as better for maintaining normal blood pressure than one 30-minute session. Nice in theory. But difficult in practice since I live in a region of the world where summers are very hot and winters cold.

In summer only early morning walks are tolerable. In winter often no time of day is tolerable to be outside, especially since I suffer from Raynaud's that makes it difficult for me to tolerate cold. The solution I found was to buy a non-electric treadmill (you power it by walking on it) that would fold up and, standing, take up only a small place in a closet (and would also fit under a bed). I could watch tutorial videos for a variety of subjects while I exercised.

The treadmill has worked out well. But when I began working on this book, I would become so involved in my work, I would forget to exercise. Soon I was not sleeping as well and my energy level sagged. I told myself, "Look, if Diane de Poitiers could get up and take a cold bath and then ride three hours on horseback through the forest for exercise and come back and tell King Henri II how to rule France, you can tear yourself away from that computer and do three short sessions on the treadmill." Now that I am back exercising, I feel and work much better.

Exercise is great, but you also need to elevate. The feet and legs, that is. One of the simplest and easiest things you can do to prevent leg problems related to circulation is, whenever possible, elevate your legs. That is why In my house every chair has a footstool or ottoman. Though it is recommended that you elevate your feet while working at a desk, I have never been able to make the this work, not with footstool, ottoman, pile of books, or box when I am working at my big desktop computer. Though I did spend $50 on a very well designed lap desk that I can use with my laptop computer when seated in one of my Indian rosewood chairs (based on the design of the thrones of the Mughal emperors) and my legs on a cushioned ottoman. This folding metal lap desk also works in my wide wicker chairs. The chair seat must be sufficiently wide to accommodate the desk width, and a chair with arms are necessary to keep the lap desk from sliding sideways.

But for serious elevation, I do a session on my slant board, actually a slant bed. When I read *Cellulite: Those Lumps, Bumps, and Bulges You Couldn't Lose Before* by Nicole Ronsard, I decided that the slant board she recommended would be a help for my circulatory problems. For a a couple of decades I used one my son made for me. But after I moved to my current house, the place I needed to set it up was at the opposite end of the house from where I had to store it. Besides setup had always been laborious. I decided to spend $350 and buy a dedicated slant bed since I used one regularly.

In the three years I have used the Newton Slantbed, both the dense foam interior and the poplin cotton cover have held up well. Folded down into its storage formation, the Slantbed measures 36 inches long 15 high and 21 inches wide (91 x 38 x 53 cm) and fits nicely under my big coffee table (with its leg elevators inserted). Pulling the bed out and opening it to the Slantbed position takes less than a minute.

The company also makes a larger version of the Slantbed for those over six feet tall. For maximum small storage space requirement and portability there is also an inflatable version (about $150) that has a built in air pump that can be operated by hand or foot. All three of these slant board/beds are safer than those inversion tables/boards that you strap yourself on and hang upside down. Those inversion tables terrify me.

Slant bed breaks can revive beautifully. Despite putting a large area of my half-acre property in ground cover, vast expanses of turf require frequent mowing here at Provence-sur-la-Prairie. In the long grass-growing season, after an hour and a half session with my little electric mower, it is lovely to take a 10 to 15-minute break on the slant bed. After an additional hour and half session of mowing, I am usually definitely experiencing those sensations in my legs the French label *jambes lourdes*. A cool shower followed by a massage with one of the gels especially designed for relieving heavy legs symptoms revives me and helps my veins that otherwise might be popping.

At any time of the year, if I am feeling tired mid-afternoon, a 30-minute nap on my slant bed will revive me. Not only is a slant bed good for circulation and the legs, but many women have found sessions on a slantbed combat facial wrinkles.

As much as I love my slant bed, I realize that not everyone who would like to avail themselves of this therapy can fit the version I now use into their budget. I looked for less expensive DIY alternatives. The goal is positioning your feet about 14 inches (35 cm) above your head in enough comfort that you can spend at least 10 minutes in that position and enough stability to be safe. An ironing board with one end propped up on books or a box was too narrow for comfort and lacked stability. I tried a trundle bed with one end lowered. Unfortunately just as I got comfortable, the lower end slipped out of its notch. The pop-up was so violent it almost launched me toward the ceiling. A long lawn chair with the front legs folded down kept tipping to one side, plus the height of the chair's legs were not right for the needed elevation.

From a dealer specializing in aids for foot and leg problems, I ordered a $70 foam bed leg wedge with an undulating top that was supposed to better conform to legs than a wedge with a flat surface. I would have needed calves the size of soccer balls to fit into the top grooves. Actually with a couple of small sofa cushions, I find this leg elevator very comfortable when used on a mat on the floor or on a bed. But you can get the same elevation of legs at about half the price from one of those bed wedges used by acid reflux sufferers and a small cushion. They come in a variety of sizes to accommodate better your particular height. You place the higher end under your knees for a comfortable bend. At the $35 to $50 price point most have a zipped cloth cover. They are small enough you can store them under the bed, or in a closet. For a no-cost leg elevation you can lie on the floor and hook your knees over the seat of the sofa or an upholstered chair.

Chic French women also wear compression stockings on long flights—and often in winter under pants—to prevent vein problems. Lately I have seen a lot of colorful one-size-fits-most compression stockings for sale. To make sure you get the benefits from compression stockings you must take your measurements and buy stockings designed for your height and calf size. Every company that makes compression stockings has their own sizing. Follow their instructions for taking your measurements and picking the proper size. Best to take your measurements in the morning. Legs sometimes swell during the day. And of course you should buy two pair so you will have a pair to wear while the other is laundered.

Support stockings are energy-savers for women who must work on their feet. A nurse practitioner friend thought the panty hose version that gave support to her whole leg worth every penny. She said they made an incredible difference in her comfort standing all day doing exams. At the end of the day she was much less tired.

What about those speciality treatments that chic French women use to give a special tuneups to their legs? You do not find as many dedicated *instituts des jambes* as previously. But specialized leg treatments are offered at many of the *institutes de beauté* and spas. The *Institut des Jambes* logo still says Paris, though the institute is now located in Rennes, principal city of the Brittany region. The institute still specializes in the three leg therapies that I wrote about in the first edition of *Toujours*: *Pressothérapie, Frigibas* and *Cellu M6*. They also now offer *VIP Millenium* described as electro stimulation under infrared light.

Pressothérapie in which two thigh-high booties apply an undulating pressure to the legs for a 30-minute treatment and *Frigibas* in which chilled wet stockings impregnated with a special hypothermatic liquid at put on the legs, have been around since at least the 1970s when Linda Dannenberg wrote her *The Paris Way of Beauty* book. *Cellu M6* is a treatment in which an aesthetician using a handheld device applies rolling, suction and massage to the skin. The idea is to increase circulation and break down unwanted fat cell deposits. In the first edition *Toujours* I describe in detail a young French woman's experience with Cellu M6.

On the *Institut des Jambes Rennes* website is an account by Virginie of her experience at the institute with the *VIP Millenium* treatment. First electrodes are attached to the thigh bulges (what in the USA we call saddlebags and the French call *les culottes de cheval* (horse pants?) and the knees and stimulate these areas for 25 minutes producing a sensation of *picotements et chatouilles*, tingling and tickling. Virginie says that it is possible to lose up to 4 cm in waist and hips in less than half an hour with this treatment. She does not say whether she actually did so.

After the 25 minutes of electro stimulation, an ultrasound machine warms the legs in the same places the electrodes were attached. This is to break down the fat cells. Following the ultrasound, comes a 30-minute manual oil massage of the legs. Virginie sums up her experience with the *VIP Millenium* : Happiness!

Another specialized leg treatment you currently find offered to chic French women is an Ayurvedic massage *Pagatchampi*. Ayurvedic medicine is traditional Hindu medicine that treats mind and body and focuses on disease prevention and wellness. You find *Pagatchampi* offered in French institutes of beauty as well as in spas dedicated to Ayurvedic treatments.

Massage Vichy located in the French spa town Vichy explains that *Pagatchampi* is a strong, dry massage applied to the legs. You do not need to undress for this massage. You wear a light cotton or linen gown that covers you, but does not impede the work of the hands doing the massage. *Pagatchampi* is done on the ground or the floor for maximum benefit. A 30-minute session is normal.

Though Ayurvedic massages are available in many cities in the USA, all seem to offer the oil massages that are done directly on the skin. When I lived in India, I had no experience with Ayurvedic massage, but a certain age friend had a very positive experience. In her late 40s, she was beginning to suffer circulatory problems (largely from no exercise) that manifested itself in dark bruises that occurred from even light pressure on the skin. The physician she consulted recommended massage. An Indian woman, a masseuse, came to the house weekly for several months to do massage. The bruising problem cleared up. My friend was so energized that she enrolled in an Indian classical dance class.

Chic French women drink a number of herbal teas and infusions that offer some benefits against vein and cellulite problems. Bilberry, butcher's broom, sweet clover and blackcurrant are among the traditional teas. I particularly enjoy blackcurrant tea for its berry taste. In the USA where there is more influence from Chinese traditional medicine, teas from ginger, Chinese hawthorn, and Ginkgo biloba are drunk to improve circulation.

As for supplements, horse chestnut is one most often recommended to support good circulation in the leg veins. You can also take a Leg Veins Support Blend of six herbs known to be good for circulation: horse chestnut, butcher's broom, cayenne pepper, dandelion, prickly ash and grape seed extract. Grape seed extract alone in capsule form is also highly recommended to support leg vein health.

The special gels, lotions, and creams chic French women massage into their legs usually contain plant oils long known to be beneficial for legs. Any *pharmacie* in France will offer a large assortments of products for leg beauty and to combat *jambes lourdes* and promote vein health. The luxury skin care lines feature at least one or two speciality leg care products targeted for veins and *jambes lourdes*.

In the USA, two products that I mentioned in the first edition of *Toujours* are still available. Dr. Hauschka Revitalizing Leg & Arm Tonic is a "botanical blend of rosemary and essential oils invigorate and tone your body while minimizing the appearance of varicose veins and cellulite." The peppermint, menthol, and witch hazel in the budget-priced Burt's Bees Peppermint Foot Lotion make it equally good for legs as for feet. One you can spray on your legs is For Feet's Sake Tired Foot & Leg Spa Mist with witch hazel, spearmint, rosemary, peppermint and eucalyptus.

In the slightly under $30 range is Mama Mio Lucky Legs Cooling Leg Gel that uses a blend of menthol, aloe vera, spearmint, chamomile and yarrow. At the same price is Origins Leg Lifts that revives tired legs with menthol, cypress, peppermint and cedarwood.

If you want a Made in France product designed especially for *jambes lourdes*, the Dermstore has Decleor Aroma Dynamic Refreshing Gel. Be warned this gel contains several kinds of artificial color. Another French product offered is Guinot *Gel Jambes Legeres* Soothing Gel For Legs. This gel contains a long list of chemicals in addition to the natural ingredients.

For the most natural and budget-friendly lotion for your legs, you can mix your own of essential oils in a carrier oil base. The ingredient lists for the commercial leg products can inspire you in the ingredients you choose. General guidelines for preparing your own mixtures from essential oils are: use a 2% dilution (12 drops essential oil for each 1 fl oz (30 ml) of carrier oil for general massage oils.

For treating a specific condition such as the veins on the legs, especially when treating an occurrence of "heavy legs," you would use a 3% dilution (15 drops essential oil for each 1 fl oz (30 ml) of carrier oil). A note here that in some of the recipes for mixing essential oil preparations you find on various blogs and websites, the carrier oil measurements will be given in tablespoons. But all tablespoons in all countries are not the same. So in this book for clarity I use fluid ounces (fl oz) and milliliters (ml). The website for Mountain Rose Herbs has good information for making your own products from herbs and essential oils.

You absolutely should not apply any essential oil directly to the skin. And you should wear protective vinyl gloves to protect your hands when you are working with these potent oils. I repeat: You must dilute essential oils in some carrier oil or gel before applying to the skin. Anyone pregnant or breast feeding should get medical clearance before using any of the essential oil creations. You will also find this use warning on commercial preparations for legs.

When I set out to mix my own leg lotion from essential oils, I immediately encountered what I call The Peppermint Puzzle. In Dr. Hauschka Leg & Arm Tonic, in Burt's Peppermint Foot Lotion, in Tired Foot & Leg Spa Mist, and in Origins Leg Lifts mentioned above, products designed to treat "heavy legs" and prevent or alleviate spider and varicose veins, peppermint is an ingredient. And a touted ingredient. Yet when I looked at various information on mixing your own essential oil leg massage lotions and gels, I found the warning that peppermint oil was not to be used by those who suffered from high blood pressure.

On none of those commercial products I checked was there any warning about use by those with hypertension. Though some products did carry the warning against use by pregnant and breast feeding women. I had certainly not found a hypertension warning in any of the many articles in French women's magazines that recommended the use of these products designed for leg vein health. Yet certain age women were both more likely to suffer varicose veins and hypertension than younger women.

A survey of the ingredient list of French products designed for leg problems ranging in price from budget to expensive turned up something interesting regarding The Peppermint Puzzle. In no product I checked was peppermint oil listed as an ingredient. Instead the products contained menthol. Peppermint is a cross between spearmint and water mint. Menthol is one of the more than 40 distinct chemical compounds found in peppermint oil.

Also interesting was that no French product I checked contained rosemary, another essential oil for which you find a warning against use by those with hypertension. Yet you find it in several of the American leg products mentioned above. An ingredient that appeared in most of the French products was arnica. You will see it also listed an *Arnica montana*. This herb grows in the USA and Europe and has been used since at least the 1500s to treat muscle pain and to reduce inflammation. Arnica is used in homeopathic medicine. If you want to use menthol in place of peppermint oil in you leg concoction, you can purchase it from some vendors who sell essential oils. At the time of this writing, Mountain Rose Herbs sells menthol crystals that have been extracted from corn mint.

So whether you want to save money or to avoid peppermint oil and rosemary in some commercial products, it is a relatively simple process to prepare you own massage oil for legs. The ingredients and process I chose came from information I read on the The Herbal Spoon, Mountain Rose Herbs, and on the well-designed and informative Think Oily website created by Vancouver, Canada, manual therapist Sally Wong who picks up tips in Chinese medicine in visits to her grandmother in South China.

To create my own leg lotion, I used 5 drops each of the essential oils of cypress, cedarwood, and lemongrass (all highly recommended for leg vein problems) mixed into 15 ml each of jojoba oil and grapeseed oil. To this I added ¼ teaspoon (25 drops) of Vitamin E oil that would serve as a preservative. Because I was mixing only a small trial amount of the lotion that I would use quickly, the Vitamin E oil was really not necessary. The mixture produced a massage oil with a silky texture and woodsy fragrance that reminded me of Weleda's Birch Cellulite Oil.

Since I save things I think might be useful (and save me money I would have to spend buying them) I had washed out and saved some 2 fluid ounce amber glass bottles with glass droppers in which I the liquid stevia I buy had been bottled. Amber glass is not absolutely necessary for your essential oil mixtures, but it is advised. While mixing, I did wear vinyl protective gloves to prevent accidentally getting any of the undiluted essential oils on my skin. I also put the cats outside. After my calico Kiri jumped up on the bathroom counter as I was preparing to brush my teeth and managed to flick her tail into the toothpaste I had just squeezed onto my toothbrush, I try to prepare against any bizarre pet eventuality. In addition to pets, it would also be a good idea to keep undiluted essential oils out of the reach of children.

One French method for applying the leg lotion is described in a *TopSanté* article *Jambes lourdes : 3 techniques pour détendre vos jambes*, Heavy Legs: 3 techniques to loosen your legs. Loosen in the sense of improving circulation. The first technique assumes that you are having an attack of *jambes lourdes* and you need to cool your legs down immediately. In that case, the first step is the cool water spray technique on the legs that I described previously in this chapter.

The second technique is the massage itself. You should plan on about 2 to 3 minutes for each leg. This leg massage is done seated—on a bed, the sofa, the floor, even the bathtub when all the water has been drained out. You will need to assemble your lotion or gel for your legs, a towel to protect the bedding or carpet from accidental spills of lotion, and some method of timing your massage such as your smartphone or kitchen timer. Or just a clock. Since you will want to elevate your legs immediately after the massage, you may want to have a cushion handy for your back or feet.

Seated on the bed or sofa or whatever place you have chosen, bend your legs so they form an inverted V and place your feet flat. Put a small amount of lotion or gel in your palm and apply it to your legs from the ankle to your thighs. Then start your timer and, beginning at the ankle, do a gentle massage to the knee. Go back to the ankle and massage again to the knee. Remember you must always massage toward the heart. When you have completed the massage on the time you have chosen, repeat the process with the other leg. This massage can be done with your own or a commercial leg product.

It seemed strange to me that the *TopSanté* leg massage instructions as well as others that I checked on French magazine websites, gave instructions to massage from ankle up to and including the knee— some toes to knee. If the massage was to alleviate the burning, stinging sensation in the thighs you have with *jambes lourdes*, why not massage the thighs also? And spider and varicose veins appear above the knee as well as below.

Whether you massage the whole leg or only to the knee, you must take care you do not put any pressure on any spider or varicose veins. These veins are already damaged. You should not stress them.

The third technique is elevation. This might be just remaining seated for another 30 minutes or so with your legs stretched out in front of you. Perhaps reading or watching television. Or it might be that you want to stretch out and elevate your feet higher than your head and take a nap. Or you might do this massage immediately before bedtime and go to sleep after the massage.

But what if you don't have time for all this spray, massage, elevation? Especially if you aren't in the midst of an attack of *jambes lourdes*? Another version of the leg massage appeared in a *Femme Actuelle* article, *Jambes légères : 3 astuces à adopter,* Light Legs: 3 tricks to adopt.

Do regular massages. Take your ankle in your hands. Place the thumbs on the back of the calf, then go [massage] straight up to the inside of the knee. Then perform some pumping movements with both hands on the back of the knee. Press for 5 seconds, then release for 5 seconds. Do the same movement in the groin to stimulate the lymph nodes to reboot the eliminatory system.

If all this sounds confusing and complicated (as French techniques often do) just massage your legs for two and a half minutes each leg. In five minutes you are done. Whatever version of massage you do, it will be necessary to do it every day. You will likely not see any visible results for six weeks to two months.

Preventative measures can help, but sometimes there comes a point where herbal teas, leg gels and creams, massage, treatments by *institutes de jambes* or spas, wearing compression stockings during long flights, elevating legs are not enough. When leg problems become severe, medical treatment is necessary.

THE MEDICAL OPTIONS

Fortunately, today, for severe varicose veins problems there are more treatments than stripping the veins. I remember how my mother-in-law who had the procedure described stripping in such unappealing terms.

Today we have a choice in treatments. In sclerotherapy a solution (Polidocanol or Sotradecol) is injected into the vein causing it to fade and eventually disappear. For certain kinds of varicose veins there is a version of sclerotherapy in which a microfoam is injected into the vein. In France this is called *la sclérose à la mousse* which sounds to me rather like a dessert on a restaurant menu. Radiofrequency ablation works when a small catheter is inserted in the vein and heat produced by radio waves causes the vein to seal shut instantly.

A new treatment for varicose veins that only received FDA approval for use in the USA in February 2015 is VenaSeal. In this minimally invasive treatment that requires no anesthesia, a "glue" is injected into the vein to seal it. No need for wearing after-treatment compression stockings, and the patient can return to vigorous exercise almost immediately. VenaSeal had a demonstration on the Dr. Oz Show. You can find videos of the procedure (and other varicose vein treatments) on the Internet.

The only vein treatment that I have experienced personally was having a nest of broken veins on my right leg treated by laser. The treatment was acceptably effective, but only a small area could be done in that treatment. I was annoyed at the clinic because the technician failed to provide me with information about after-treatment procedure so I did not have on hand the necessary supplies and I did not get as good results as I would if properly prepared for immediate after-treatment care. From this experience I decided any future vein treatment would best be done in a medical vein clinic and not in place that specialized in cosmetic procedures.

FASHIONS FOR LONGER, LEANER LEGS

Chic French women are never satisfied to just look good, they want to look sensational. Because they put such high priority on attractive legs as key elements in their appearance, they don't just put out effort and money for leg care. Keep in mind that most chic French women are not tall. Most chic French women do not have exceptionally long legs. They just know some style tricks to make their legs look longer and slimmer than they actually are.

Inès de la Fressange, tall with exceptionally long legs, is often touted as an icon of Parisian style. But her mother was a South American fashion model. Former French first lady Carla Bruni Sarkozy, also tall, and like Inès, a former fashion model, was born in Italy of Italian parentage. One reason current French first lady Brigitte Macron makes a good French style icon is that she comes from a long line of native French, and her height (about 5 foot 4 inches, 1.64 meters) is more typical of French women than the mostly foreign-born fashion models you see in the Paris runway shows.

Footwear News, a publication of the shoe industry, analyzed Brigitte Macron's shoe style choices to make her legs look longer and leaner. I found amusing that the magazine commented that the French first lady usually chose "sensible heel heights, usually no more than 4 inches." Generally one inch or one and a half inches would be considered "sensible." But we live in the era of 5 inch stilettos, don't we?

The magazine wrote: "Macron has an athletic, thin figure and styles herself in a way that complements her appearance. She avoids T-strap sandals that cut off the ankle and can cause some people to look shorter than usual; instead, her preferred shoe silhouette is a pointed-toe pump, which can help create the illusion of extra height." Rounded toes make your legs look shorter. The writer adds: "Some of the shoe styles she wears include statement-making accents such as PVC material, metallic hardware, cutouts, cap toes and snakeskin—all fresh touches that give a classic look an energetic twist."

Brigitte Macron uses other chic French style tricks to make her body look slimmer as well as her legs look longer and leaner. For my analysis, I am using dressing for longer, leaner legs information provided by *Stylecaster*. For instance, Brigitte Macon often wears monochrome outfits in darker, neutral colors. With the exception of the open-toed burgundy sandals she wore in Italy with slim white jeans, she usually matches her pant and shoe color, another way to give a longer, slimmer body line. And boots with a v-shaped top cut are a more-flattering transition from legs to feet. This is particularly good for very petite women. For women with exceptionally short legs, wearing high-waisted pants with the top tucked in gives the appearance of longer legs. Also pants in dark colors with longer inseams (high-rise, high waist) give an appearance of a longer leg. I would add that they are generally more comfortable than pants with shorter inseam. Many women wearing pants with high waists certainly look more attractive when viewed from the back.

My height is a shade under 5 foot 4 inches (1.6 m) and my legs shorter than most other women at this height because my neck is unusually long. Factoring into these body proportions, my mid-70s age, I find the most flattering style is for pants with straight or wide legs. Pants tapered at the ankle, especially tight-fitting ones, accentuate my short legs and widen the appearance of my thighs.

Additionally I avoid cargo pants. (Except some excellent quality 100% cotton ones I bought at a bargain sale price that I wear for mowing the lawn because they are so comfortable in the heat.) Even if I do not put anything in those side pockets of cargo pants, just the zippers, stitching and extra fabric seem to make my legs look shorter and wider. And I never buy pants with elastic in the waistband. Even if the elastic is only at the back, the bunching of the fabric makes my hips look broader—and my legs fatter and shorter.

In analyzing Brigitte Macron's spectacular legs, interesting to note that almost every article on legs in French women's magazines cautions that wearing tight-fitting pants and high-heeled shoes will cause unattractive leg problems. Yet tight pants and high heels are two major elements in Brigitte Macron's personal style—and the personal style of many chic French women who, like Brigitte, have spectacular legs.

While I have never seen any scientific studies that shed light on this conundrum, it seems obvious that all these products and treatments I have written about previously in this section work sufficiently well to offset any problems that the tight pants and high heels might cause. Also this caution against the tight clothing and high heels originated in a day when fabrics did not have the engineered stretch that can prevent putting undue pressure on certain areas.

Too, today shoe designs are better than in previous times. One reason that chic French women favor very expensive shoe lines is not just the style factor, the shoe designers are very talented shoe architects who can design wearable and walkable shoes at high heel heights.

CHIC CERTAIN AGE LEGS

Not long after the inauguration of Emmanuel Macron as president of France, *Vogue* published a short article focused on the French *Première dame's* legs titled "Brigitte Macron's Jaw-Dropping Legs Prove That, in France, Age Is Just a Number." The article commented:

Aside from being 24 years her husband's senior, at 64, Macron's favorite unconventional fashion choices feature hemlines that fall well above the knee—and place her gamine, toned, and tan limbs squarely in the spotlight. But lest one think Macron only shows them off for official occasions, the First Lady left her home in Le Touquet-Paris-Plage on a bicycle in June clad in a crisp button-up, sneakers, and a denim miniskirt that hit at mid-thigh. Historically, the French have never set an expiration date on femininity or sensuality. This may explain why, at a time when America's youth obsession is paramount, and its restrictions on women ever-more pervasive, Macron's rejection of outdated age- and gender-related dress codes feels particularly remarkable. Visible on a global scale, France's First Lady is cutting a liberating new feminist path with her particular brand of Gallic body confidence. In politics, as in life, what could be more powerful?

Age *is* just a number. And with the right techniques and products such as those discussed in this chapter, certain age legs can be just as beautiful as those of younger women. Brigitte Macron's legs certainly prove this is true.

Feet

A SHOCK. WHEN I SAW PHOTOS of chic French women, icons in the French fashion industry, wearing gleaming white sneakers on their chic French feet, it was a shock. How many decades had the fashionable French looked down their chic French noses at "sneaker-wearing Americans?" What was it they called white sneakers and running shoes? Marshmallows, wasn't it?

A definite transformation has been taking place in French chic in recent years. Fashions for both men and women are receiving an infusion of the more casual styles that have long been common in other countries, especially in the USA. When I returned to live in the USA, in my French-influenced style of dressing I would show up for an event in a dress and heels. Almost everyone else would be wearing jeans—or a track suit and running shoes. Even for concerts.

Athleisure is wearing clothing and shoes designed for workouts and sports for leisure-wear or social functions. Or even to the office. Athleisure was a strong fashion trend among the chic French in 2017. It shows no sign of fading in 2018. In footwear, top designers are offering more sneakers and athletic shoe styles—and boots with thick low (and high) heels replacing those thin stiletto heels.

Of course when chic French women wear sneakers, they wear streamlined styles, often very expensive brands of sneakers. Hundreds and hundreds of euros per pair. And chic French women wear those expensive sneakers in very chic French ways. In the summer of 2017, for instance, I was seeing Paris street fashion photos that showed the flat streamlined white leather sneaker worn by young French women with white, full-skirted, almost to the ankle length dresses. Note that monochrome dressing in which the shoes match the clothes elongates the body line making the wearer look taller and slimmer.

This trend for sneakers and for pumps and boots with thicker heels does make it easier for certain age women—French and others whose personal style is influenced by French chic—to wear more comfortable shoes and still look "in style." Especially when they must walk long distances, this is helpful.

From the time we learn to walk, for most of us, our feet do their job without much difficulty: they take us where we want to go and— without much coddling— they wear those styles that complete our chic. But then, about the time we reach certain age, our feet turn cranky.

When a woman reaches certain age, her feet may begin to develop bumps, toes may crook or draw up, spurs can sprout on heels, ankles sometimes sag one way or the other. Walking while wearing chic shoe styles is not always as easy as it once was. Then one of two things likely happens. Neither of them advisable.

Unfortunately, too many certain age women use foot problems as a reason (excuse?) to be less active than they previously were. And too often with that reduction in physical activity comes weight gain that makes walking on problem feet even more difficult.

The other response of many certain age women in the USA to developing foot problems is to give up their high heels and sexy, feet-flattering shoes. They begin wearing flat, "sensible" shoes that sabotage their chic personal style.

Vanity can also cause serious problems for certain age feet. Too many women are so proud of their dainty little feet that, when in certain age,

those feet need a bit more space for comfort, these women refuse—
absolutely refuse—to buy a larger size shoe. This makes walking misery
even in shoes designed for walking.

Shoe companies have not (thank goodness!) gone in for ego-
sizing the way clothing makers have, but still not all shoes made by all
companies labeled a size are the same. Buy the shoe that fits, whatever
the number that the company has stamped on shoe and shoe box. But
be aware too that it is not always a larger shoe size that is the solution to
the foot problem. Too large shoes can cause problems just as too small
ones. The goal is shoes that fit properly and comfortably whatever the
style or heel height.

Of course, chic French women don't give up their stylish shoes in
certain age. First lady Brigitte Macron and other celebrity chic French
women of certain age and their footwear are positive evidence of this.

But how do chic French women of certain age overcome those
problems that propel American women to "grandma" shoes?

Valérie Jardin is a French-born, USA-based professional photographer
currently living in Minneapolis. She hosts a popular street photography
podcast *Hit the Streets*. Valérie Jardin regularly takes students to Paris
for street photography workshops. Street photography is photography
that captures candid, unposed scenes in public places such as parks,
cafes, and streets, usually when the subjects are unaware they are being
photographed. Street photography invariably involves a LOT of walking.
It also demands the photographer blend in with people in those public
places. In Paris, that means footwear that can keep you comfortable and
yet be sufficiently in style that you don't stand out as a tourist.

On a *This Week in Photo* podcast focused on travel, Valérie Jardin
explained to host Frederick Van Johnson the advice she gives to her
students preparing for one of her Paris workshops. Her recommendations impressed me as excellent advice for any woman of certain age

who wanted to wear stylish shoes and still walk comfortably. Whether in Paris or in her own city.

Since Valérie Jardin's students must "hit the ground walking," first of all, she advises that they bring two pair of in-style, well-broken-in shoes. Good shoes, are, of course, expensive, though they can be resoled to stretch their years of service. Valérie Jardin admits that since she is constantly leading street photography workshops in Paris (and other major world cities) she usually spends more in a year on footwear than on camera gear. But she cautions that the best-made stylish shoes will surely require inserted insoles for comfort for long sessions of walking.

Valérie Jardin also advises students to bring a supply of blister pads for toes and heels—and apply them at the very sign of discomfort to prevent a blister from becoming a debilitating problem. She likes those thin pads that slip over the blistered toe like a new layer of skin.

True French woman that she is, Valérie Jardin would not, when questioned, reveal the specific brands of shoes she buys for all that street photography walking—though she did confide that she buys European brands. I would agree that, generally, in European brands you can find a shoe comfortable for walking that is not actually a walking shoe—nor does it look like a walking shoe.

As for blister pads and inserts, it is hard to beat good old Dr. Scholl's for wide selection and quality. Well-designed, affordable, and available almost anywhere. If you are unsure which product is best for your foot problem, on the Dr. Scholl's website there is a products page on which you select your particular problem and click. You are then shown the products designed for those problems and given an explanation of the differences in them. By the way, Dr. Scholls makes a special insert for your dressy high heels higher than two inches.

Band-Aid also makes blister pads and other products to heal your foot problems. A number of companies make those slip-on gel toe sleeves to prevent blisters. If your local stores do not offer these foot savers, they are easy to find in online stores. Make sure you buy the correct size for your feet.

Of course, your feet are going to be happier if your shoes have been "broken-in" to accommodate their particular vagaries, especially if you are one of those many people who have one foot a slightly different size than the other. When you were younger, simply wearing shoes for short periods of time until they molded to your feet would usually do the trick for adjusting to your feet. Certain age feet may require more.

I had an uncle who always wore custom-made cowboy boots. Even though these boots was made specifically for his feet, he always put the finishing perfection on their fit by filling his bathtub with about six inches of warm water, then standing in the water until the leather was well soaked. Then he would wear the boots until they dried and they would have stretched in places needed to accommodate his feet. I thought this was loony. Until . . .

One morning I was caught in a rainstorm waking wearing a pair of Calvin Klein heels. I had not had time to break in these dressy shoes very well and they were still uncomfortable across the toes. But that rainstorm day, I had no second pair of shoes with me and did not get home until late. I had to wear those wet (and slowly drying) leather shoes all day. The next time I put them on, they fit perfectly. Uncle's system worked.

Shoe repair shops—if you can still find one—can make adjustments to your shoes to make them more comfortable. Or you can invest in shoe stretchers. The longer durability of the wood and steel ones usually make them worth their cost. Keep in mind that stretchers for flat shoes may not work with high heels or boots. Those may require special stretchers. You can also buy gadgets that stretch out a small spot to accommodate a bunion. But try to wear shoes that fit well enough that you won't develop a bunion. Or a corn. Though I understand corns are easier to deal with. A good podiatrist can be a help for more serious problems that drugstore pads and inserts can't help.

The regular services of a good podiatrist who can provide a medically-based pedicure for prevention of foot problems are another way chic French women are able to avoid certain age foot problems.

Useful here that I remind you of the basic foot care advice of Paris "foot guru" Bastien Gonzalez, an *artiste de la pédicure*, that I outlined in the first edition of *Chic & Slim Toujours*. After bathing, always dry toes well to prevent fungal growth. (I always give my toes a finishing touch with my hair dryer on warm to get my toes totally dry.) Massage the feet nightly, especially the fatty cushion at the bottom of the foot to keep it supple and bring back its volume. This is especially important if you wear high heels every day. I was given as a gift some lovely lavender foot cream that I use in winter. I think it actually helps keep my feet warmer. In summer sandal weather I like a lavender foot balm.

That leg massage I described in the previous Legs chapter will also help circulation and minimize foot pain. In addition to the leg massage, Bastien Gonzalez also recommends that, if you wear very high heels, each evening do calf stretches and pull toes forward to relieve pressure on the joints.

If there was any doubt in my mind that French attitudes were changing toward footwear, there on the cover of May 2017 French *Elle* was the pretty blonde wearing a gauzy strapless print dress pulled up to show her crossed knees and her chiffon petticoat—and her unlaced white leather sneakers. One thing I noted was that in recent French chic, often the wearing of sneakers seemed to demand fuller, longer skirts. Visually these balance the bulk of the shoe. Though you also often saw sneakers worn with skinny jeans.

Then, on the September 2017 cover of *Elle* there was certain age Juliette Binoche dressed in a one of those slightly baggy pant suits some chic French women have lately been wearing. And Juliette was barefoot.

Surely younger French women can look chic in sneakers and clunky boots, but what about certain age women of more advanced years? I wasn't sure until I saw an image that settled the question in my mind.

The black and white photo was one taken by photographer Valérie Jardin on her summer 2017 visit to Paris. An older couple, perhaps in their 70s, are walking hand in hand along a Paris street and are looking at the displays in the store windows as they walk. He carries a parcel and a small shopping bag. She carries a small neat shopping bag and her handbag is over the shoulder. Her hair is worn in a sleek gray shoulder-length bob. Her winter jacket is thigh length and her straight skirt comes conservatively below her knees. She is wearing dark opaque tights with white leather sneakers. Comfortable chic casual for certain age.

Not all chic French women are willing to give up their ultra high stiletto heels in certain age. The former editor-in-chief of *Vogue Paris* Carine Roitfeld is an example. Carine, though now 63, maintains her signature style of heavy black eyeliner, pencil skirts and ultra-high stiletto heels. She has only disdain for sneakers. As she told *The Guardian*: "I would never buy sneakers. I really dislike them! I dare you to find a picture of me wearing sneakers. I don't wear them. I think it is unattractive."

Keep in mind that this disdain for sneakers expressed to *The Guardian* came after three back surgeries and time in a wheel chair and a back brace necessitated by a fall in New York the year previously. Carine Roitfeld told *Vogue* in February 2015: "I had an accident one year ago in New York. I fell down and I broke some bones, and you know because I am always running, I do not always do what I need to do. And finally I had an operation, and after one operation I had a second operation, and after the second, I had a third operation."

In the original *Chic & Slim: How Those Chic French Women Eat All That Rich Food And Still Stay Slim*, I wrote: "A French woman would prefer to have her legs amputated rather than be seen in clunky exercise shoes." Perhaps I should update that to: "A chic French woman of certain age would rather have three back surgeries and spend time in a back brace and a wheel chair than be seen wearing sneakers."

Even so, today we certainly are seeing many chic French women of certain age wearing sneakers, the chic French first lady among them. Chic French footwear styles are changing.

Whatever style shoe you choose for your certain age personal style, treat your feet with kindness by maintaining a healthy weight. If your feet are not carrying a heavier load than that for which they were designed, they will likely work more efficiently and look their prettiest.

Hair

CHANGER DE TÊTE. In French, the phrase for change your hairstyle translates literally "change of head." When certain age launches changes in your hair, you often need a *changer de tête.* Almost certainly you will need different products and care techniques than when younger. But out of the overwhelming number of choices these days, which?

As in personal style, skin care, and weight control, chic French women can be useful role models to help us make *changer de tête* choices. Additionally a number of dedicated Paris-based coiffeurs are working to develop techniques and products and generously sharing their expertise so that we can put them in practice no matter where we live—or whether our budgets allow for their pricey services and products. Can't afford top Paris colorist Christophe Robin's Cleansing Purifying Scrub with Sea Salt for your hair, he provides you with the DIY recipe. More advice from Paris coiffeurs further into this chapter, but first a look at the chic French approach to hairstyles and hair care. Then, we will look at why many of these chic French approaches are especially beneficial for certain age hair.

David Mallett is a scruffy, outspoken, but nonetheless charming hair stylist transplanted from his native Australia to Paris via Italy and London. In the past two decades he, in his eccentrically, but elegantly decorated Second Arrondissement salon has earned the reputation as a wizard of haircuts. His ability to turn a head of fine limp hair into one with volume and bounce has made him the choice of models and actresses and huge numbers of chic women. With his Paris headquarters and international clientele, David Mallett has observed various approaches to hair care and has been forthcoming in interviews (with Noël Duan for Yahoo News and Kathleen Hou for The Cut) on the topic of French women and their hair. So what attitudes, techniques and products create the current version of chic French hair?

First of all, according to David Mallett, chic French women want their hair to have an "undone" look. You find this look described in French fashion magazines as *le coiffé-decoiffé naturel* look, the styled messed-up natural look. In any case, it means their hair does not look as if a woman has spent all afternoon and an obscene amount of money at the hairdressers. According to David Mallett, "French women will put in so much effort to look like they didn't do much at all."

Also French women wash their hair only every five to ten days and consequently don't strip out natural oils the way more frequent washing does and requires a conditioner to replace. According to David Mallett French women can do these less frequent shampooings because they are less *"sportif"* and don't require an after-workout shampoo. I would add that generally French women do not have the problems with excessively oily hair that many American women do. Then there is summer heat. In the USA, women don't have to be *"sportif."* They can work in the garden, take their children or grandchildren to the park, or just sit outside in hot weather and find themselves with perspiration-soaked hair.

As for chic French women of certain age, David Mallett says that they will give up trendy hairstyles they have worn in their 20s and 30s and go for classic hairstyles that suit their personal style. "Nothing makes a woman look older than stiff blow dry. It makes them look like robots. Hair has to have life and movement. French women are connected to life. [Their hair] doesn't have to be perfect. But no frizz. Anything frizzy and dry is unacceptable."

An example of a chic French woman who wore trendy in her 20s and 30s, but chose classic in certain age is Michèle Alliot-Marie (71), the former Defense Minister, who also served in several other French cabinet positions. The *dame en fer* "iron lady" has in certain age worn a classic short cap of natural gray hair with side part and swept to the side bangs. Yet in a slide show on the French *Vanity Fair* are 15 images of a younger Michèle Alliot-Marie with very feminine shoulder length waved blonde locks—a look more starlet than French cabinet minister. Though both styles incorporated attractive eyeglass frames.

French women also avoid over-layering. David Mallett suggests, instead of layering, a cut with thick edges and only a little thinning out on the ends. Also more subtle highlights done with *balayage* instead of foil highlights. Or perhaps a transparent color wash [glosses and glazes] that makes their haircolor appear more subtle and subdued. Over-brushing is also avoided. Instead, finger combing leaves the hair a bit tousled.

No matter whether short or long, colored or natural, one thing all chic French women want in their hairstyle is low maintenance. That means a haircut that does not require frequent trimming. It means hair color that lasts months, not weeks.

Why this emphasis on low maintenance? The current state of the French economy is a factor. Many women, especially women 18 to 30, who as a group are burdened with 25 percent unemployment, just don't have much money to spend on hair products and services. Also Mathilde Thomas, co-creator of the Caudalie skin care line, says French women want low maintenance hair because they devote so many hours to skin care that they don't have much personal maintenance time for their hair.

Caroline de Maigret, one of the authors of *How to Be Parisian* explained the insistence for low-maintenance in an interview with Harper's Bazaar:

> It's the self-confidence to feel that you're okay without adding more. It's more chic. Refinement and elegance are in details, rather than opulence and showing off. But we don't want people

to think that we take too much time doing futile or frivolous things. If you arrive with a lot of the hair and makeup, that means you wasted that time while you're supposed to do something more interesting.

As for more interesting things to do, Caroline de Maigret (43), in addition to her regular jobs of model and music producer also works on women's education projects with CARE, an international humanitarian organization working to fight global poverty.

Christine Lagarde's (61) job as director of the International Monetary Fund demands frequent travel. Her short cap of silvery gray hair is the perfect choice for her demanding schedule and choice of swimming for her exercise. Since the previous edition of *Chic & Slim Toujours*, Christine Lagarde has married Marseille businessman Xavier Giocanti. A new husband certainly rates as more interesting than complicated hair care.

Françoise Bourdin (65), the fourth bestselling writer in France, also wears her hair in a short blond cap. Hers is gold-toned with side part and bangs. An immensely practical style for a woman who writes bestselling novels year after year—but who still must look chic in interviews promoting her books.

Audrey Azoulay (45), is a former French culture minister and new director general of UNESCO. The French civil servant often wears her shoulder length dark hair in a profusion of natural curls framing her face. Other times the curls are clasped low at the back of her head. Both styles offer easy maintenance for someone facing the arduous task of revitalizing a troubled organization to fulfill its original purpose of protecting "the world heritage of humanity."

Christiane Taubira (65) is a former French Justice Minister who is more recently—along with Paris mayor Anne Hidalgo and former French Social Affairs Minister Martine Aubry—founder of the new *"mouvement d'innovation" Dès Demain* that aims to promote social democracy, the environment and active citizenship. Mme Taubira's very practical hairstyle is a neat coil of braided hair at the base of her head. I well understand the low maintenance of this hairstyle because my grandmother wore her hair, that she never cut in her entire life, in the same sort of braided coil. Instead of the neat rows of braids across the top of the head that Christiane Taubira wears, my grandmother, who had very straight hair, clipped metal clamps onto wet hair that dried into Marcel waves.

Fleur Pellerin (44) France's former minister for small and medium-sized enterprises, innovation and the digital economy, is currently a businesswoman working to promote France's tech industry with her venture capital firm Korelya. A Korean orphan adopted by French parents, Fleur Pellerin wears her dark straight hair in a short bob with side part. From her photos that appear frequently in the media, you can see her hairstyle is an excellent example of how chic French women can space their haircuts many months apart. The style can be cut short to a length above the chin. As it grows down to shoulder length, it continues to look sleek and professional. For formal occasions, Fleur Pellerin sometimes adds curl giving the haircut a softer, more feminine look.

Noëlle Châtelet (73) has the naturally curly hair so many of us envy. An occasional trim, and if desired, some haircolor. *C'est tout!* Mme Châtelet parts her hair in the center and lets the dense curls form a blonde aureole, the circle of light around the head in paintings of saints. This low maintenance hairstyle is perfect for her busy life as prize-winning novelist and non-fiction author, university lecturer (she wrote her PhD thesis on eating disorders), and advocate for death with dignity.

Whether you go high or low maintenance, at some point in certain age you likely will find that, for health, financial, or lifestyle reasons, the haircut that served you so well so long, just no longer works. The good news is that so many of the world's most skilled hairdressers are now sharing their techniques via internet videos that any hairdresser anywhere can learn those techniques. You have much better chance of a really good haircut even in small towns and rural areas now than even a decade ago. But, of course, you have to put out effort to find those skilled hairdressers. Unfortunately, you may have to endure a bad haircut or two before you find them. Fortunately, hair grows back.

HAIRCOLOR OR NATURAL

Once you decide on your certain age haircut, you will have to decide about color. Will you go with natural or haircolor achieved by single-process, double-process? Or semi-permanent, permanent, highlights, low-lights, glazes, glosses? You have choices between chemical haircolor or the newer plant-based haircolors now becoming more available, especially in Europe. And there has long been the gray hair solution henna—with all its flaming orange advantages and disadvantages.

Whatever hair color modifications that you choose, you must be cautious that the changes don't themselves announce aging. Think of those women who at the first signs of gray hairs begin applying a dark flat haircolor that does not harmonize well with their skin tones and actually makes facial lines more noticeable.

On the other hand, covering your gray in a way to maintain your hair color as it grays can give an impression that you are not aging. A woman I have known since childhood is a natural blonde. As she has grayed, her hairdresser has cleverly colored the gray so that her hair color has remained the same as when she was pre-gray. She takes good care of her skin. Now in her late 70s, she doesn't seem to have aged.

Up until several decades ago a few gray hairs, the "silver threads among the gold" were seen as a natural part of aging. But today, because so many women disguise even the first sprinkling of silvery strands, a bit of gray is less acceptable. Note the reaction when the Duchess of Cambridge, then age 33, was photographed with a few gray hairs showing. (Since she was pregnant at the time there was good reason for not applying haircolor chemicals.) An uproar ensued in the media and on social media. Catherine's gray was quickly covered.

On the other hand, when American actress Diane Keaton arrived at the 2014 Golden Globe awards with her gray hair in a long bob with chunky smoky silver lowlights over pearly white, her hair was seen as the ultimate in certain age chic hair. Journalists and social media praised the haircolor. Professional colorists wrote articles analyzing the technique that produced the lowlights.

Total gray will be applauded as "embracing your natural gray" But just a few gray hairs showing will be considered ill-groomed. So what do chic French women do at the first signs of gray?

In the past, French women's first gray was often treated with henna. The powdered dye made from the dried leaves of *Lawsonia inermis*, also known as mignonette tree or Egyptian privet is inexpensive and easy to apply. Reportedly henna does not wash out. Ever. Depending on the natural haircolor and texture of the hair to which it is applied—and the henna paste mixture used—results produced may be a pale orange to a deep auburn. In any case, a warning: you absolutely cannot put henna on your hair if it has any sort of haircolor treatment on any part of the hair. And if you have put henna on your hair, any hair treated with henna must be totally cut away before you apply chemical haircolor.

Since so many French women have not altered their naturally dark hair, henna over their gray strands usually gives a deep auburn cast and creates a haircolor that I call French certain age mahogany. Yet according to top Parisian colorist Christophe Robin, Parisian women coming to his salon today want no mahogany. He told *Elle* US in March 2017 that instead they want a cooler ashy shade of brown.

A note here that at the time I wrote the first edition of *Chic & Slim Toujours*, Christophe Robin's website featured photos of famous French actresses whose certain age hair he had rendered in rich shades of mahogany with buttery *balayage*. Styles change.

French attitude toward haircolor is definitely different from that of Americans and offers benefits for certain age hair. In considering the differences, keep in mind that certain age brings hormone changes that makes hair dull, flat, and brittle with a tendency toward thinning. When hair grays, it becomes more fragile and more susceptible to damage from chemicals and heat appliances. It is more likely to break when stressed.

In an April 2017 interview with *W Magazine*, titled "Christophe Robin on What Americans Can Learn From French Women About Hair," the colorist summed up the French approach. When asked what he thought were the biggest differences between American and French women with haircolor, he answered: "I believe in America you do a lot of gloss every five minutes. You wash your hair so many times, and you oxidize your hair so many times, that it's like putting more makeup on the dry skin, you know?"

But a French woman will likely spend much less time on maintenance. "A French woman is going to spend time on the weekends taking very good care of her hair to have very low maintenance with hair color." Good care, Christophe Robin insists is going to mean less effort daily.

For treating those first signs of gray, Christophe Robin prefers to do a *balayage*, the painted-on highlights, because it is easier to camouflage that scattering of gray hairs. As for covering hair that is totally, or at least mostly gray, Christophe Robin believes the single process color should get a light highlighting. "I always try to make it look like it was a real natural color. And that's how it looks young. You think of girls like Juliette Binoche or Kristin Scott Thomas, when you start to cover your grays a lot, and just do it so many times, it becomes very dark and it turns mahogany." And that mahogany would signal that a woman is covering gray. He says, "What I try to do is to make it look like if it was your own natural hair, and like this doesn't look old, it doesn't look like you're covering your grays." Highlighting can also make hair look thicker, even if it is only one shade different from the base color.

If a woman wants to have beautiful hair—at any age—she must take care of her scalp. For a long time, women and their hairstylists concentrated on the hair, but now we understand that if the scalp has problems, it will be difficult to have healthy hair. As Christophe Robin explains, if a woman is stressed, this can cause such poor blood circulation that it results in hair loss. His remedy? "I tell them give themselves a good [head] massage upside down every night before they go to bed for three minutes. And I tell them to relax, to do yoga, to breathe, because so many girls when they're stressed, the scalp is too tense onto the bone, and blood circulation is very bad."

So how do you pick the right hair color? You aim for a color that harmonizes with skin tone and eye color that is easy to maintain on healthy hair. New York stylist Lisa Chiccine told "Oprah's Gray Hair Bible" for *Prevention* magazine that "Gray or white hair tends to look best with pink, olive, and dark complexions, If you're sallow or very pale, you'll probably look washed-out and should consider highlights or lowlights. Brown hair that looks mousy as the gray comes in can be brightened and enriched by weaving in highlights and lowlights of honey, tortoiseshell, or mahogany." Lisa Chiccine adds that if your gray comes in wiry and tends to stick up, weekly deep conditioning is going to be necessary to make it behave. No doubt the weekend hair masque application popular with French women will tame any wiry gray.

As for Lisa Chiccine's recommendation for lowlights for the very pale, I will tell you that a certain age friend had white, white hair, very light blue eyes, and very pale skin. Her son complained that since her hair grayed that her head looked "all white." She added lowlights in the reddish blond shade that had been her natural before-gray haircolor. Those lowlights took 20 years off her face. Her features were more noticeable. You were more aware of how pretty her well-cared-for skin.

One of the *Chic & Slim* readers shared photos of her transformation from brunette to natural gray with charcoal lowlights. Charcoal lowlights on silver gave her a chic sophistication that the single-process brunette color did not. They also freed her from monthly haircolor. Her lowlights only require redoing every six months. Big savings in money and time spent at the hairdressers.

If you choose the lowlights on total gray option, remember that you can always do a trial with semi-permanent haircolor to see if you like the results. This gives you an opportunity to test out various shades.

NATURAL AND PLANT BASED HAIRCOLORS
The trend in France for plant-based haircolor thrives. More hairdressers are offering the natural haircoloring—and in attractively decorated salons. The pioneer for natural haircoloring is Romain of Romain Colors who in 2002 was the first to offer natural and organic haircolors in his Paris salon.

In spring 2017 when Romain opened his new salon (in a secret location near le Madeleine) *Vogue Paris* noted that he was the first to offer haircoloring both vegan and gluten-free. The opening was covered, with photos of the elegant black and white interior of this Second Empire classic Parisian apartment, by all major French fashion publications including *Madame Figaro, ELLE, Grazia, and Vogue*. The salon, a *Club Privé*, offers its members once-a-month customized services in a *déconnecté* (no wi-fi) environment where, according to the report I read, photos and posting to Facebook and Instagram are forbidden.

Another Paris colorist who is moving more and more toward the plant-based color is Marisol Suarez at her Studio Marisol. She told *Madame Figaro* magazine that as she began to suffer from headaches and from skin damage to her hands, her concerns about chemical haircolor and its effect on both the hairdresser and clients lead her to move toward banishing products with ammonia, bleach, and chemical dyes. Marisol Suarez acknowledges that many clients are still hesitant to adopt natural haircolor because the processing time is longer and the pigments disappear from the hair in a shorter time than with chemical dyes. But she is making the option more attractive by creating easier transition from chemical to plant-based color. A strong advantage for natural haircolor is that the underlying natural color is not affected and regrowth is not so noticeable.

Another Paris salon offering plant-based haircolor is the salon *Les Belles Plantes* of coiffeuse Gaëlle Grippon. As the colorist explains on the salon's website, more style-conscious French women are abandoning flat dyes and sliced *balayages* in favor of natural and transparent coloring. She adds that natural haircolor pigments can be used to camouflage gray hairs and thinning spots and other imperfections for certain age women. For women accustomed to chemical haircoloring, the salon offers an alternative with semi-vegetable dyes that will allow a smooth conversion towards the 100% natural. One of the natural haircolors offered at *Les Belles Plantes* is the professional line NATULIQUE founded by a Danish couple Mette and Stig who explain that they became concerned about the link between health problems and today's cosmetic products after Mette was diagnosed at age 28 with breast cancer and they feared a connection to haircolor she used.

L'Oréal has also created a no ammonia oil-based permanent haircolor INOA. Other companies have developed professional lines of natural haircolor. As far as I can learn, almost all satisfactory plant-based haircolor is only available in salons. Other than henna, none of the DIY herbal rinses seen to cover gray effectively. For instance, those who have tried a sage and rosemary rinse do not give it high marks. While the sage and rosemary herbal rinse does not effectively cover gray, it reportedly does mute too-light highlights.

For gray hair with a yellow cast, women long used laundry bluing to combat the yellow. In the USA, in my grandmother's generation, women kept a bottle of Mrs. Stewart's Bluing (a colloid mixture of ferric ferrocyanide and water) on the pantry shelf. They added this bluing to laundry water to whiten sheets and put it on their hair to make their gray appear whiter.

Though chemical, not herbal, laundry bluing cannot have been too harmful. Many women in my grandmother's generation I knew who used it lived healthy lives well into their 90s. But they definitely qualified for the description "little old blue-haired ladies."

AVOIDING HAIR LOSS

Ten years ago a *Marie Claire* article on hair loss in older women stated: "We're living longer, and we're torturing our hair like never before. Combine that with increased environmental insult and basic chronological aging, and you've got an epidemic of parched, brittle, and frayed 'old lady' hair."

Of course, the "epidemic" has now been contained. In the decade since that article was published, we have become much better informed about the needs of certain age hair. The hair care industry has developed products and techniques to combat the so-called old lady hair.

First came awareness. Magazine articles such as that one in *Marie Claire* made us aware of things that we could do—and stop doing—to keep our hair thick and healthy. We were reminded we should not put tight bands on our hair, nor jerk a comb through it when it was wet. Twisting it up in a towel after a shampoo would cause breakage. We should not shampoo with extremely hot water because it would strip hair of oils and make it vulnerable to breakage. And yes, stress, could make our hair fall out. Really. But, the Mayo Clinic assures us, if we can control the stress, we can stop stress-induced hair loss.

Still more magazine articles and online beauty sources reminded us that chemical haircolor was hard on hair and to space our haircolor as much as possible. For root touch-ups we should take advantage of the greatly improved products to cover the root regrowth: sprays, or gels applied with a wand. Or even powders. Some root touch-ups work better than others.

Dermatologists reminded us that what we ate did make a difference in the health of our hair. Hair needs protein and a certain amount of healthy fats. And hair needs a B vitamin called biotin, also called Vitamin B7. And if we don't get enough biotin from brewer's yeast, soybeans, butter or sunflower seeds, we can take a supplement. Fish, poultry, eggs, beans and low fat yogurt are recommended to prevent thinning hair.

The encounter of immigrants and their traditional hair products with Parisian hairdressers gave us a whole raft of new products based on their traditional treatments. Argan oil from Morocco, coconut oil and prickly pear oil from lots of places. Australian river salt. You could buy the pricey products with these natural ingredients. Or on the Internet you could find recipes galore for DIY hair masques and oil treatments, particularly for argan and coconut oil, that would strengthen certain age hair. Appliance manufacturers designed increasingly more powerful drying and styling appliances, but we learned this greater power was dehydrating our hair when used too frequently on too high settings.

The greatest help in controlling the epidemic of "old lady hair" was the multitude of products, quite effective products, designed specifically for the needs of certain age and graying hair. Treatments were developed for inherited female pattern hair loss. Dermatologists could prescribe topical Minoxidil products specifically formulated for women and hormone replacement therapy for post-menopausal women.

Scalp massage came back in style as a way to prevent hair loss. I can testify that my mother from my earliest memory demanded a vigorous scalp massage at each of her weekly hair appointments. Her hair was as thick and shiny on the day she drew her last breath at 93, as it had been when she was a young woman.

And then on top of all the aforementioned advice we were told that certain age hair requires different shampoos and washing techniques than when we were younger. Certain age hair does not require—or tolerate—shampoo and water as frequently as younger hair. So how often should we shampoo?

My sophomore year in college, the university housing office, in what was surely the worst mismatch of the semester, assigned me as dorm roommate a proto-hippie from California. She had shoulder length naturally curly dark brown hair that she only washed every two weeks. If then. Shampooing only twice a month! Or less. I was horrified.

She thought my once-a-week or oftener shampooing habit excessive and quaint.

To be fair, her hair never looked bad, even the last days of the second week. Naturally curly hair generally is drier, less prone to oiliness than straight hair. But in early 1960s, the once-a-week shampoo was almost unwritten law. Then things changed.

For my generation and younger women, lifestyles and hairstyles made the every day or every other day shampoo a necessity. Well . . . until the hair experts began telling us that we were washing our hair too often. Lately they are telling us we are not shampooing often enough. Especially those who are spacing shampoos with a dry shampoo. Even if most of your life you have struggled with oily hair, it will become less oily in certain age. Frequent shampooing will be neither necessary nor advisable. Once every five days works for many women over 50.

Paris colorist Christophe Robin says the question he is most frequently asked is how to wash hair to maximize volume and shine and to retain haircolor. He has become such a crusader-advocate for proper hair washing that he has installed in his new Rue Bachaumont Paris salon an arty basin in the form of a giant seashell inspired by Botticelli's painting "The Birth of Venus" in which Venus with her cascade of glorious red-gold hair is standing.

For a *New York Times* article in 2017, Christophe Robin outlined the steps for proper hair washing. First detangle the hair with a good brush to eliminate stressing and possibly breaking wet hair with after-shampooing combing. Second, apply a moisturizing hair oil [almond oil will work] to the ends of your hair and leave on at least 15 minutes. The oil eliminates need for after-shampoo conditioner that can weigh down hair and decrease volume.

Third, wash your hair with a shampoo designed for your hair type. If you have color-treated hair, make sure you have a sulfate-free shampoo. Use moderation in amount of shampoo used. Too much can be difficult to rinse out. Shampoo left in hair can cause serious problems, not the least of which is hair loss.

Christophe Robin's last step is a reminder not to damage wet hair with excessive rubbing, and certainly do not twist it up in a towel (as many of us have been doing since we first began to wash our hair—and which I find an almost impossible habit to break). He suggests instead a Moroccan technique where you flip your head upside down and rub a towel over it from alternating sides. Having switched to this system (I use sweet almond oil for the moisturizing oil) I can testify that my hair does have more volume and shine than with my previous system by which I shampooed and then applied a conditioner to the ends. With both systems I use a sulfate-free shampoo for color treated hair.

What do you do when you can't for one reason or another shampoo? Instead of dry shampoo, Christophe Robin suggests adding five drops of apple cider vinegar to five ounces of water and spritzing it at the hair roots to remove oil.

Nonetheless, dry shampoo is popular in France. One preferred by French women is Klorane, a moderately-priced dry shampoo available in pharmacies. In the USA, there are a number of dry shampoos designed specifically for certain age hair. My one experience years ago with dry shampoo was such a bad experience I have never again used one. I would suggest that you if you do plan to stock a dry shampoo for emergencies, give it a trial before it is needed. Not fun to find yourself miserable with flu and your hair full of gunk you are too sick to shampoo out.

THOUGHTS ON CERTAIN AGE HAIR

In the USA, hair is such an indicator of age, especially out here in the heartland where I live. Sometimes when I am waiting at the salon for my haircut, my hairdresser is finishing up another certain age customer at her weekly appointment. I struggle to keep an expression of horror off my face as curling iron wraps the client's short, chemically-colored, dry and frizzed by its permanent wave, hair. I try not to grimace at the extensive backcombing. I hope not to be too obvious as I dive to a far corner of the room so as not to inhale the cloud of hairspray engulfing us as the setting product is applied.

Why do these women subject their hair to such torture? I wonder. My hairdresser does excellent haircuts. Why don't these women let her cut an easy-to-maintain style that can be air-dried and given a quick touch with a warm curling iron with no potentially damaging permanent waves, backcombing, and heavy hair spray necessary?

Years of habit are difficult to change. I understand that. But healthier hair and looking more youthful and attractive might be worth it.

Caroline de Maigret, one of the authors of *How To Be Parisian*, told *Harper's Bazaar* that the strongest indicator that a woman was not French was her hair. Caroline de Maigret believes that if a woman can get the hair right, she is halfway to looking French.

I would add that chic French hairstyling and maintenance techniques will result in attractive, healthy certain age hair that will cost you less time and money to maintain.

You certainly will avoid having "old lady hair."

Face

FRENCH AND AMERICAN certain age women respond to signs of aging on their faces differently. Very differently.

For a long time, in their attitudes toward those physical changes, in their choices of skincare products and procedures, and in their expectations for the results of various treatments, the difference was as great as between a *boulangerie* baguette and supermarket sliced bread.

But the differences are not as great as previously. Much has changed on both sides of the Atlantic in recent years. Certainly we have seen the adoption of new products and techniques—and the revival in popularity of several traditional ones—in both France and the USA.

Still, one can generalize that American women want their anti-aging efforts to make them look young. French women want theirs to make them look attractive. American women start their corrective treatments at the first signs of aging. French women begin their anti-aging efforts in their teens.

When a wrinkle appears on an American woman's face, she wants it banished. French women are more blasé and tolerant about the signs of aging. At least the current generation of French certain age women are. But I am not so sure that the French women who are now in their 20s and 30s will share the same tolerance as their mothers and grandmothers.

Nonetheless, Mathilde Thomas, founder of the French skincare line Caudalie and author of *The French Beauty Solution* sums up the difference: American women see beauty treatments as quick fixes. French women see beauty treatments as long-term investments in their appearance.

These days French women's magazines are filled with anti-aging articles—and many are careful to point out that there is a difference in treatments that are *anti-rides*, anti-wrinkle, and those that are anti-aging (for which the French use the same words as in English). You see many anti-aging articles, but only a few *anti-rides*. Many anti-aging articles are aimed at women younger than 40, rather than older.

In any case, French women spend a reported ten percent of income on skincare. What is that money buying these days? Which of these treatments and products to which French women are so devoted might be most useful for women—like most of you reading this book—who do not live in France?

The good news is that almost all the treatments and products popular in France today are available in the USA—and in many other countries as well. Though, usually, outside France they cost more.

FACIAL MASSAGE

Facial massage has long been an important part of French facials. The idea is that the face is underlaid with muscles, and when these muscles lose their tone, signs of aging appear. Just as the muscles in the other parts of the body need exercise to maintain their tone, so do the muscles of the face. Many women accomplish this tone maintenance with facial exercises, making those prescribed weird contortions in a daily workout. I tried facial exercises in my 30s, but found the expressions they created disturbing and the results disappointing. Instead I continued with a light facial massage I had already incorporated into my daily evening cleansing routine. Of course, facial self-massages in no way equal the massages done by a skilled practitioner. That is why the best facial massages cost you hundreds of dollars per session.

In her article on facial massages in *The Financial Times*, Vicci Bentley described the French style:

> Deep, kneading *petrissage* enlivens and tones the skin; rhythmic, butterfly-light *effleurage* relaxes and boosts lymphatic drainage; stimulating *tapotement*—firm but gentle taps and slaps—invigorates sluggish circulation and muscle tone. A dextrous repertoire of pinching, cupping, rolling and rocking is designed to sculpt, recontour, tighten and decongest.

In any list of current top practitioners of facial massage in Paris, you will find the names of Joelle Ciocco and Biologique Recherche's *Ambassade de la Beauté*. Biologique Recherche is a French skincare company that makes a line of skincare products popular in the USA including the Lotion P50 with its cult-like following.

Joelle Ciocco and Biologique Recherche represents opposite approaches to French facial massage today. Joelle Ciocco is all-manual. She foregoes any of the high tech machines that have been incorporated in facial treatments of late. Biologique Recherche, however, combines traditional manual massage with microcurrent treatments and even uses a high tech device to create nanofiber hyaluronic acid patches which are placed on the face and dissolved.

The original French facial massage was based on a system devised in Sweden in the 1800s, but today facial massages available in France have incorporated techniques from many areas of the world. Some practitioners specialize in treatments that use massage techniques from Japan or North Africa, the Orient via California, or India. Even the Amazon area of South America has provided techniques.

Martine de Richeville in her Facial Remodelage program incorporates Chinese medicine. This fully manual treatment is done on the whole face including eyelids and neck. Stroking, palpating-rolling and lymphatic drainage are all employed to help the face regain its ability to defend against environmental toxins and to slow down the signs of aging.

A type of facial massage enjoying a renaissance in France are the *Jacquet pincements*. I first learned these facial pinches in *Christine Valmy's Skin Care and Makeup Book* when I was in my late 30s. This Romanian-born woman who pioneered the profession of aesthetician in the USA recommended Jacquet massage to help control excessively oily skin. Her instructions included no information on how long these pinches were to be performed each session, only:

> Apply a night-treatment cream. Lightly pinch the thicker portions of your facial skin between thumb and forefinger and rotate the flesh in a half turn. Do this until you have covered all the fleshy parts of your cheeks and chin. To remove the excess oil that has been expressed, dip a cotton pad in cold water and lightly tap your skin with the soaked pad. Pat your face dry.

Today in France the Jacquet pinching technique developed by a French doctor in the 1930s to treat scars and other wounds of war is used to combat wrinkles, acne and blackheads, rosacea, light scarring, bags under eyes and signs of fatigue, also to promote blood circulation and better oxygenation of the skin.

The best information in English about use of *Jacquet pincements* in France I found was on the website of the French skincare company Christian Breton. Instructions there are simple: "On clean and dry skin, pinch the skin between thumb and forefinger with rapid gestures to reach the deepest muscles."

In a *Votre Beauté* article listing practitioners offering various sorts of anti-age facial massage in Paris, two were identified as offering the Jacquet pinching: the salons of Galya Ortega and that of Annie. The latter is particularly enthusiastic about Jacquet massage. *Votre Beauté* says after a 60-minute session with Annie that:

> Her clients also note better tissue oxygenation. The complexion loses dullness, is clearer, pinker. Puffy faces are refined, the drainage of the bags under the eyes is spectacular and, over

the course of the sessions, rejuvenating and anti-wrinkle effects assert themselves.

AT-HOME DEVICES

Chic French women have been slower than American women to incorporate at-home devices into their facial skincare. Aesthetic services for the face are much more widely available in France. Even small cities and towns have their *instituts de beauté*. Training of aestheticians is far more rigorous in France and standards for certification higher than in the USA. Even so, prices for facial services in France are generally less expensive than in the USA.

Yet French women have shown such interest in at-home devices for replacing or topping off professional treatments between sessions that French *Elle* recently suggested two devices in their *"7 astuces pour paraître plus jeune dès demain,"* 7 Tricks to Appear Younger Right Now. The Carita My C.L.E. is described as:

A device that works on the firmness, the uniformity of the complexion, and the brightness of skin. It combines microcurrents to stimulate the muscle fibers of the skin, with LEDs, which stimulate cell activity and optimize the benefits of care.

The second device mentioned in the article was the Philips' VisaPure Advanced, a 3-in-1 facial treatment device that is similar to the Clarisonic Cleansing & Micro-Firming Massage device. Carita is a French luxury skincare line with an extensive product line for anti-aging. At the time of this writing, the Carita My C.L.E. seems to be available only in the EU. But we in the USA have a growing number of popular at-home devices.

None of these at-home devices, of course, equal the facial treatments of microcurrent, LED or radiofrequency performed using the higher-power machines used by professionals in salons. But many users feel these at-home versions give sufficiently satisfactory results that justify their multi-hundred dollar prices. Plus they offer anywhere-you-are use, eliminating expensive salon visits that often involve fighting traffic and then interminable waits for the technician who is invariably running behind schedule.

At the salon you might have Thermage to strengthen and stimulate your collagen and elastin production and to lift and tighten the skin. But the same radiofrequency technology is utilized in the NEWA Skin Care System device for home use.

Many LED treatments are available at salons and medispas these days. For at-home use, the LightStim For Acne uses red and blue LED lights to heal existing blemishes and reduce future breakouts by eliminating acne-causing bacteria. The Baby Quasar Clear Rayz also uses blue and red LED technology to clear your complexion and prevent future breakouts. The Baby Quasar Plus Light aims at reducing lines and wrinkles.

The companies that design these devices are constantly introducing newer and more powerful models. The devices I mention in these pages may have been discontinued and replaced with improved ones by the time you read this book. Some general guidelines regarding them should be followed for any purchase.

Town & Country magazine published an in-depth look at LED at-home devices. From it we have these takeaways: First of all, the LED technology in these at-home devices is sound science. The US National Aeronautics and Space Administration developed it in their research on healing in space. Power is important when choosing a device. You need at least 500 watts per square meter (W/m^2) to stimulate collagen production. Battery-operated devices likely will not provide you with acceptable results. You need a device that plugs into an outlet. Blue lights treat acne. Red lights treat signs of aging. Treating acne will probably be more effective with the devices that combine red and blue lights. I would add that the combination of red and blue lights would certainly seem preferable for certain age women still struggling with breakouts and who also want to combat lines and wrinkles.

Microcurrent technology is widely used by top facial salons in both

France and the USA. Biologique Recherche uses it extensively their facials in France. In the USA, top facialists Joanna Vargas in New York and Los Angeles and Joanna Czech in Dallas, use this technology as a part of their celebrity-favored massages.

In the line of at-home devices that use microcurrent technology to give instant results of a lifted toned appearance, the current queens (and princesses) are the NuFace devices. NuFace even offers a mini version that you can carry in your handbag. If you are looking a bit fatigued, you can whip out your NuFace Mini and give yourself a five-minute facial.

After reading a jillion articles, reviews, and product descriptions for these gadgets in research for this skincare chapter, I have reached several conclusions that might be useful if you are considering buying one.

First, these devices offer treatment benefits to those who, for various reasons, cannot avail themselves of the salon versions. For those who do pay for the expensive salon versions, they can extend the benefits of those salon treatments, in some cases making possible longer intervals between salon sessions.

Second, these devices do get results and are safe—when they are used as the manufacturer specifies. American users must simply avoid the too-common more-is-better mindset. On the other hand, users should not expect results if they do not use the devices as often as directed and in the manner directed. Some devices require gels or add-on equipment. And sometimes these add-on pieces you must buy separately are almost as expensive as the device itself.

Third, the devices work as part of a personal skincare program that includes other non-device elements: your cleansers, peels, serums, etc. No one should expect that they would use the device and dispense with all other skincare and get results. At-home devices are unlikely to achieve the results of injectable fillers.

Fourth, if you are going to invest in one of these many devices, spend time on research before you make your choice. For some who have not previously used these devices, the wealth of information can be dizzying. Take your time.

Fifth, buy directly from the device company or its authorized reseller (often resellers offer better prices) and make sure that the seller offers a money-back return policy. I was happy to note that some of these devices come with a 30-day, some even with 60-day, return policy. Every salon treatment I ever had required that, before the treatment, I sign an agreement that even if the procedure did not work as advertised, I still had to pay full price for it. Several times they did not work—and I still had to pay full price for them. The money-back guarantee that comes with most of these at-home facial improvement devices seems to me a definite plus in their favor.

SKINCARE PRODUCTS

Much of the world's most sought-after and expensive skincare products are made by French companies. And some of the world's most effective and budget-friendly skincare products are sold from the shelves of French pharmacies. You don't have to be affluent to buy good skincare in France. French pharmacists are knowledgeable about skincare and they regularly provide advice and recommendations to their customers as to the best products for their skin. These days via the Internet, word about effective skincare products spreads quickly globally and produces demand. Now in many countries outside of France you can buy French skincare products popular with chic French women. If not in your local department store or drugstore, certainly online.

If you read interviews with chic French women in which they disclose the skincare they use, often you will find their moisturizer of choice is *Embryolisse Lait-Crème Concentré*. Actually much of the reason it is so popular with models, makeup artists and others whose faces are so important to their success is that it can be used as primer, moisturizer and makeup remover. On the product page of Embryolisse USA, shea butter and aloe are touted as the important ingredients. In actual fact in the list that ranks ingredients by their weight in the product, water comes first, as is usual in cosmetics. Second is *paraffinum liquidum*, a highly refined version of mineral oil used in cosmetics. Shea butter comes eighth on the list, and aloe is 14th out of 18.

Always interesting to me to note that some primary ingredient in a product that French women find so useful, is on the avoid list in the USA. A number of dermatologists and aestheticians in the USA warn mineral oil will clog pores. To remember here: The company recommends *Embryolisse Lait-Crème Concentré* for dry skin. In general, French women's skin tends to be drier than those of women in the USA. Genetics, climate and other factors play roles here. *Embryolisse Lait-Crème* is an example of a product that might work well for French women—but might not get as good results for those with different genetic makeup and location.

French women like facial cleansers they do not have to rinse off with water. When I wrote the first edition of *Chic & Slim Toujours*, cleansing milk, *lait démaquillant*, was very popular, especially those milks that were natural and organic. Now the popular no-rinse cleansers are micellar waters. And these are chemicals, chemicals and more chemicals—with hardly a natural substance to be found in their ingredient list. Though the popular Bioderma Sébium does have a little Ginkgo biloba leaf extract and the Bioderma Sensibio has some fruit extracts and cucumber.

The science behind these facial cleansers is that the micelles, little particles suspended in the water that attract dirt and oil to themselves, are in the solution on your cleansing pad. As you rub the pad across your face, the micelles grab up the dirt and oil and leave your face clean. Most micellar waters can also be used to remove eye makeup. Micellar waters offer a real advantage in areas where the tap water is heavy with minerals or chemicals that dry out skin.

Now it seems that every skincare line offers a micellar water. Most offer two or three. Ingredient lists on these waters vary enormously. Prices range from budget to expensive. I have not yet become a total convert to micellar water. It is difficult for me to accept a cleansing product that does not require careful rinsing.

Once La Roche-Posay was a somewhat exclusive French skincare line. A few years ago they became more democratic, distributing their products in pharmacies in France and in the USA. While becoming more widely available, La Roche-Posay apparently did not lower their quality—nor their prices. In 2017 La Roche-Posay Toleriane Double Repair Face Moisturizer won The Oprah Magazine Beauty Award.

Another line of skincare products that have become popular in the USA in recent years are those from the laboratories of Biologique Recherche, particularly their Lotion P50 Original "1970." I mentioned Biologique Recherche previously when I wrote about their use of microcurrent technology in their facials—in which they also use their various lotions. I first read of this exfoliating, skin-balancing product in an interview with an aesthetician who uses that Biologique Recherche lotion in her facials. She mentioned the skin-balancing was provided by the apple cider vinegar the lotion contained. Curious as to what else went into this expensive and much-lauded lotion, I searched out an ingredient list. When I read that one of the ingredients in P50 Original "1970" was phenol, I had to smile.

Another name for phenol is carbolic acid. When I was a child, my grandmother liberally dispensed an all-purpose medicinal salve she mixed herself. The only ingredient in this salve that I can remember, other than the white petroleum jelly base, was carbolic acid. Despite the ecstatically satisfied users of P50 Original "1970" who claim it has made near-miraculous improvement in their faces, some women are still leery of the phenol and opt for one of Biologique Recherche's milder lotions without it. As many of my cuts and scrapes my grandmother doctored with her homemade salve, I can assure them that, if phenol in a product was dangerous, I would never have lived to age six.

Chic French women have never been as obsessive about sunscreen use as American women. But France is considerably further north of the equator than the USA. Sunlight there is not as intense as it is in the USA, especially in the southern portions. Personally, I have never accepted the prevailing belief in the USA that ultraviolet light rays from the sun should be totally avoided. Note the word totally.

When I was a teenager suffering badly from acne, my mother sent me to the best dermatologist in our area who, every two weeks, would lower a gigantic sunlamp within millimeters of my nose and sunburn my face. This was the high tech treatment for acne in those days.

While I was writing this skincare chapter, in a conversation with a cousin in Oklahoma City who suffered acne in her early 20s, she reported that she went every other day on her lunch hour to her dermatologist's office where she had the same type of ultraviolet light treatment.

In those days, magazine beauty articles recommended sunlight exposure for clearing acne, with home sunlamp treatment in the winter months. I wore out one sunlamp and used the second for years. In addition, a good part of my adult life I lived in locations with the beach right out my back door providing frequent sessions of sun exposure. For years we received all that "sun is good" advice, and then overnight medical opinion on sunlight changed.

No longer was sunlight beneficial for Vitamin D production and strong bones and the way to clear up acne by drying excess oil. Sunlight would give you skin cancer and age your skin so you would look like a stale raisin. We were told we must wear sunscreen all day every day.

I think you could accurately describe my use of dedicated sunscreens over the past years as occasional. All the brands I tried, even the very expensive ones promised not to clog pores, caused my face to break out. Of course, sun protection is included in many serums, moisturizers and foundations, so I have had their protection. Also, in certain age, I have followed the pre-sunscreen prescription of no sun exposure after 10 AM nor before 4 PM. If I must be outside in the sunlight in those prohibited times, I wear a broad brimmed hat. I do use sunscreen on my arms and shoulders if I think there is danger of a burn. Throughout my life, I have often tanned, but I was always careful avoid sunburns. Too painful.

Because sun exposure and proper means of protection from ultraviolet rays is important, I was interested in two comments on sunscreens that I read in my research for this book. One comment was made by the head of a skincare company, a woman who also oversees numerous skincare spas worldwide. The other was by one of the top facialists in the USA.

Mathilde Thomas was born and grew up in Grenoble at the foot of the French Alps. Today she is co-creator and co-owner of Caudalie, the French luxury skincare company whose products harness the anti-aging power of resveratrol in grapes. In an interview with US *Vogue*, Mathilde Thomas was asked what products she would recommend bringing back to the USA from visits to France. She responded: "I would bring sunscreen, because we have better sunscreen in France. Any sunscreen is better [than in the U.S.] because of the regulation."

The magazine article did not clarify to what the regulation Mathilde Thomas was referring. But one assumes it was one of our Food and Drug Administration regulations whose specifications render various French products less effective. One example is L'Oréal's Elnett hair spray which, according to Kathleen Hou of *New York Magazine*'s The Cut, the French version can be brushed out and is a favorite with top French hairstylists. The version you find on the shelves of American stores and those ordered from American vendors, to meet FDA regulations, is a product that cannot be brushed out. I have no idea what the difference in American and other countries' sunscreens. But I trust that Mathilde Thomas knows what she is talking about.

Facialist Joanna Czech was born and trained in aesthetics in Poland. For many years resident in the USA, she has treated her impressive celebrity clientele in her salons, first in New York and now in Dallas where she lives. From her photos one can see that Joanna Czech has that lovely light Northern European skin. And since I live not far from Dallas, I have often observed how hard the Texas sun can be on lovely light Northern European skin. Additionally the facialist is in her 50s and says the amount of time she spends flying for business is hard on her skin. In an interview with the beauty-focused website *Into the Gloss*, when asked about sunscreen, Joanna Czech said:

> For SPF, no more than 15. The one I use daily is Clarins, but on the beach I'll go for Environ's 25 or La Mer's 30. I've been paying attention to certain studies—I was at a lecture several years ago from a chemistry professor at UCLA and she talked about how some SPF 50s involve so many more chemicals, and can cause more bad than good. That's why I try to stick to 15. I do chemical sunscreen, not mineral. I do believe in a certain level of chemical in my sunscreen.

Added to skin concerns about ultraviolet rays, now air and water quality have been added. *The Financial Times* quotes Dr. Stefanie Williams, medical director at London skin clinic Eudelo:

> Until recently, excessive sun exposure was thought to be the main environmental hazard leading to premature skin ageing. But more and more studies are revealing that urban pollution is just as harmful, leading to increased wrinkling, loss of elasticity and irregular pigmentation.

Before we all retreat to an isolated mountaintop in Tibet, we should take comfort that skincare companies are developing products they have dubbed "toxic avengers" to deal with that urban pollution threat.

FRENCH SKINCARE PROTOCOLS

Whether they buy budget skincare products at the *pharmacie* or pricey ones at an upscale spa, chic French women observe certain skincare protocols.

First, chic French women believe that too aggressive cleansing can do as much harm as not getting the skin properly clean. Morning cleansing involves splashing with cold water, preferably a mineral water friendly to skin. Some skincare companies sell atomizer or spray bottles of mineral water with or without herbal additions for facial cleansing.

Many American women (myself included) who have tried this French morning splash of water find that it is simply not enough to cleanse our faces of oil and nighttime-acquired impurities. Breakouts and clogged pores result. Still it may greatly improve your skin if you can determine the least amount of morning cleansing and with what products that will leave your skin healthy without creating other problems.

Second, chic French women believe that hot, even warm water, on the face is to be avoided. Whatever touches the face, should be cool or cold. Writer Anne Bauso tracked down the science behind why cold water is better for the skin. She interviewed dermatologists Joshua Zeichner and Judith Hellman for an *Allure* magazine article. The doctors explained that hot water can strip the skin of essential oil that protects the outer layer. When the skin's lipids (or fats) start to wear away, moisture creeps out of the gaps in your skin's barrier. The skin develops cracks, can't properly protect itself, and further loses water content. And if that wasn't bad enough, hot water dilates the blood vessels and can result in flare-ups of rosacea and other skin problems.

Third—and this is a kind of golden rule—before sleep the face must be absolutely clean. No matter how tired they are, chic French women know that good skin requires that it must be absolutely clean before they apply any nighttime treatment and retire. That is why, as their lives become busier and more complicated, these women want effective cleansing products that work thoroughly and quickly.

Fourth, chic French women give attention to their eyebrows. They may skip the eyeliner, give the barest touch of mascara to lashes, but their eyebrows will be well defined. In addition to facials, Joanna Czech's salon offers brow services. The Dallas aesthetician whose business has long been faces reminds us: "There are many practical reasons why eyebrows are the most important facial feature we have."

When certain age brings thinning eyebrows to our faces, we should not neglect to become skilled with correcting this deficiency on this important facial feature. Some eyebrow gels contain volumizing fibers. If thinning becomes excessive, there is "permanent makeup," that is, tattooing. Or eyebrow extensions in their various manifestations. You can have a technician apply hairs one by one to create fake brows in a salon. The thinner your brows, the more expensive the process. But salon eyebrow extensions are an excellent way for those who have lost their eyebrows in chemotherapy to regain their brows immediately.

For those who want regrowth of their natural brow hairs, there are various eyebrow serums. According to dermatologist Joshua Zeichner quoted in a *health.com* article, to foster regrowth, the serum must contain peptides. One product that seems to work well is RapidBrow Eyebrow Enhancing Serum.

If you want to spend about a $1000 and undergo a certain amount of pain, there is microblading where pigment is implanted under your skin with a manual handheld tool instead of a machine. Recovery time is uncomfortable for many and touch-ups are usually necessary.

THE SKINCARE AGE

In 1995 film version of Jane Austen's novel *Persuasion*, Anne Elliot in a conversation with Captain Wentworth's poetry-obsessed friend Captain Benwick, says of the early 19th century in which the story is set: "We are living in a great age for poetry."

Shelley, Coleridge and the rest of the Romantic poets are long dead. No one would say that today we are living in a great age of poetry— though perhaps one could make the case for texts and Twitter messages. But no one would deny that we are living in a great age for skincare.

Never before in the history of the world have there been so many products, so many treatments, so many devices, so many medical and aesthetic practitioners devoted to making our faces look better than our genetic material has designed. And the Internet makes possible near instantaneous information about all these products, treatments, devices and practitioners. Never before have women, looking in the mirror and seeing signs of aging, had so many ways of making those signs vanish if they have the desire. And the money.

So, overwhelmed as we are with all the possibilities, we must decide how much of this improvement we will avail ourselves. Appearance is important, but how much intervention in Nature do we need to be happy and successful? The answer will be different for each woman. You have to work it out for yourself.

One last thought: Chic French women believe their appearance is important. They devote much time, effort and money to making their faces attractive. Yet they believe that, in the long term, a well-cared-for face with the natural signs of age is better than a face that too obviously looks as if it "had something done."

Eyes

WHAT GRIEF OUR EYES can give us when we reach certain age. Oh dear! Fortunately medical and cosmetic science have come up with a large arsenal of techniques and products to deal with both vision and appearance problems our certain age eyes present us. Many of these techniques and products work very well—though the ones that correct our vision and erase those age signs best are usually the most expensive.

Still, you do not need to be rich to see well and have more youthful looking eyes in certain age. But you do need to know your options—and the pros and cons of each—to help you make the best decisions. New products and techniques are continually developed. Much new has appeared since I wrote the first edition of *Chic & Slim Toujours*.

In certain age, properly corrected vision is not an optional luxury. To move about safely and to appear chic, it is a necessity.

Think of those certain age women you have seen whose makeup is, let us say, awry. Foundation not spread evenly, blush like clown cheeks, eyeliner smudged and uneven, lipstick out of line. In the blur of their faces in the mirror, to them everything appeared lovely. In certain age to put on makeup well you need adequate vision, adequate light, and a good magnifying mirror. Don't neglect those three. If you can't see how you really look, you can't really look chic.

In that first edition of *Chic & Slim Toujours*, I wrote about my adventures with presbyopia and reading glasses. You can read about those adventures in that book. For this book, I will tell you that I still remain totally enthusiastic about multifocal contact lenses. I wear them except for long sessions working at the computer or reading. For those sessions I have progressive bifocals optimized for that work. I have worn those optimized eyeglasses for driving or walking short distances. But because they are optimized for about 26 inches (.66 m) from my eyes, they make objects and the ground seem closer than they actually are. I believe that I can walk and drive more safely wearing my multifocal contacts. My supposition on this matter was reinforced when a friend who wears trifocal eyeglasses told me that in city traffic she grazed the side of a truck. She says through her eyeglasses it appeared that her vehicle was adequate distance from the side of the truck. But it wasn't.

Until certain age, I had wonderful 20/20 vision. In hindsight, I realize those beginning certain age years when I relied on reading glasses were unnecessarily difficult. If I had it to do over again, I would have shortened the time I depended on reading glasses and moved sooner to a monovision system. In the earliest stages, I might, as President Ronald Reagan, have worn one contact to correct for reading and left my still-good distance vision uncorrected. Then, when it became necessary, to wear a contact lens in one eye corrected for distance and the other for reading. On the other hand, the chief reason for depending on non-prescription readers so long was that much of that time my budget required the more economical solution.

Especially in certain age, finding the right eye doctor is important. Very important. You can waste money paying for eye exams from doctors unwilling to accommodate your need for chic as well as how you want your corrective lenses optimized. The first eye doctor I dealt with wanted a compromise between work at the computer screen and driving. So both the correction for the eyeglasses and for the contact lenses were not as good as they could have been.

The second doctor (who told me he had recently hit a cow in the road because he did not see it !!) understandably insisted on optimizing both my multifocal contact lenses and eyeglasses for driving. Considering that I spend about 200 hours at the computer for every one I spend driving, this was not helpful. Finally I have found a doctor who understands and accommodates my needs for work and lifestyle. Thus, I have fewer headaches, both physical and metaphorical.

Bifocal's noticeable line used to be a telltale sign of advancing years. But they seem to have been almost universally replaced by progressive bifocals that look the same as the corrective lenses younger people wear. Progressive bifocals do cost a bit more than lined. But when it comes to looking youthful in certain age, progressives are worth it. Many who have worn both the older version and the progressive say their overall vision experience is better with progressive lenses. When it comes to trifocals, apparently the progressives win without question.

But if you do wear eyeglasses, invest in a good brand of lens cleaner. Smeary eyeglass lenses certainly detract from chic. Worse, they interfere with vision. In choosing a cleaner, remember non-glare coating for which you paid extra requires alcohol-free cleaner. Carrying lens cleaner towelettes in handbag or tote will keep your eyeglasses chic when you are out and about.

Somehow when I solve one problem, another pops up. When I finally found an eye doctor who would optimize my correction as I wanted, during my eye exam, he made the off-hand comment. "By the way, I am seeing some small cataracts in both your eyes." Oh, rats!

I have advice on cataracts, their prevention and corrective surgery, but let us take a break from the vision department of certain age eyes and look at options for dealing with those eye changes that symbolize certain age: crow's feet lines, droopy eyelids, pouchy skin, and dark circles under eyes. That unfortunate stuff. At the end of that discussion, I will return to cataracts.

MORE YOUTHFUL LOOKING EYES

For my age, 73 at this writing, the lines at the corners of my eyes are not bad. Two things I began doing back in my mid-20s slowed their development. Under the influence of French women, I began using my first anti-wrinkle cream (French *bien sûr,*) at age 25. Because I have always spent a lot of time in the sun, I have always worn sunglasses with UV filters. By my mid-40s, I began using an eye-cream, a product specifically designed for the area around the eye. Drooping eyelids have only become a problem noticeable since about age 70 — and unfortunately, the droop is lopsided, far greater droop on my left side than the other. For the bags and circles under my eyes the cosmetic industry keeps coming up with better treatments. So I keep reading the reviews and trying new products that show promise.

As you can tell from the above, my approach to the signs of aging around my eyes is very much that of chic French women: start early with sensible prevention, use a little eye cream and not worry very much about the lines and such that appear with the years.

But many women, especially American women, are horrified when they look in the mirror and see crow's feet. The want something done. Now. They want those telltale signs of age gone. If you are among them, the good news is that these days you have a lot of choices for treatment. Laser resurfacing works by boosting collagen and elastin, but the results are not what is often hoped. Something called Ulthera, an ultrasound energy that penetrates to the facial muscles, is promised to provide a non-surgical eye lift by lifting the brow. This is one of the several "targeted energy treatments:' that use infrared light, radio frequency waves or other energy forms to penetrate into the skin to boost collagen production that will smooth the lines and wrinkles.

Botox, of course, has long been the age eraser here in the USA. Unfortunately, the side effect from Botox in some individuals is drooping eyelids. Fortunately that droop is not permanent and there does seem to be a treatment to speed the correction. But the possibility of this side effect should be put into the number of factors considered in choosing between Botox that immobilizes muscles and a hyaluronic acid gel filler such as Juvéderm. These hyaluronic acid fillers, synthetic versions of a natural compound in the body, plump the wrinkles and fill in hollows.

For really wipe-off-the-years results, nothing beats blepharoplasty, a surgical eye lift. I have had three friends who underwent blepharoplasty. With two I was in email contact before and after the surgery. The third I saw frequently before and after the work. The first friend who had the surgery was a nurse of 40 years experience. No stranger to surgery, still, she was surprised by the amount of pain following the surgery, as well as by the length of time it took to heal. She was however pleased with the ultimate change in her appearance when healing was complete.

Another friend had blepharoplasty, not for appearance, but because his upper eyelids were drooping so badly that they were rubbing the outer corners of his eyes and causing irritation and vision problems. (The condition is ptosis.) Like my nurse friend, he was surprised at the amount of after-surgery pain and the amount of time it took to heal. Looking at photos taken in the first week after surgery that he emailed, it looked as if he might have been beaten in the face with a club.

My third friend had blepharoplasty as part of face lift surgery. For her, the eye lift was not as radical as might be done as stand-alone surgery. Her lesser surgical lift was to be maintained with regular use of treatments of filler. I seem to remember it was Juvéderm. This friend experienced minimal after-surgery pain and bruising. The results were lovely. Several decades vanished from her face in a couple weeks of healing. A substantial amount of money vanished from her bank account when she paid the cosmetic surgeon's bill.

L'Oréal's RevitaLift Double Eye Lift comes packaged in a small dispenser with a tube of eye cream to smooth under eye wrinkles. A second tube contains a lifting gel. Rubbing this lifting gel from the crease up to the brow gives me a lift that kicks in within an hour on this drooping left eyelid. The gel decreases the left droop to about the same amount as the slightly drooping right eyelid. Of course, if your eyelid droop is symmetrical, you can apply to both eyelids for lift on both sides.

And then there is the Karl Lagerfeld Solution for Aging Eyes. The fashion designer wears dark glasses with large lenses so that no one can see his eyes or the condition of skin surrounding those eyes. Dark glasses (assuming they have UV filters in those big lenses) also correct for glare, both a contributor to the development of cataracts and making vision less comfortable once cataracts develop.

CATARACTS

In many parts of the world, cataracts, the clouding of the normally clear lens of the eye, mean blindness or near-blindness for millions. For those of us who can afford skilled doctors, surgery to remove the clouded lens and (usually) replacing it with a clear artificial lens is not a big deal. Sometime around 1960 when my grandmother had cataract surgery, she spent several days in a hospital. Around 1990 when my mother had her cataract surgery, it was done on an outpatient basis. She cooked and served Thanksgiving dinner in her home to 23 guests two days later!

Today recovery time from cataract surgery is usually swift. Few experience problems. Still, the idea of cutting on my eyes makes me very nervous. So several months ago, when I read a headline that we might, in a few years, remove cataracts with eye drops instead of surgery, I was elated. More in-depth reading about the testing of N-acetylcarnosine by a team of Russian doctors, and the work by an ophthalmologist at the University of California San Diego with lanosterol convinced me that it was unlikely that we would be zapping cataracts with drops instead of surgery in the immediate future.

N-acetylcarnosine eyedrops can be ordered online and are available in some health food stores. If you read online reviews, these drops do not seem to be removing cataracts in either older humans or dogs very well. Lanosterol probably shows more promise for dog cataracts than human. So at the point my cataracts begin to interfere with my ability to work, drive, go about my daily life, I will need surgery. That is, unless medical science has come up with something efficient that is less invasive. We can hope.

The good news from the cataract surgery information page on the Mayo Clinic website is: In most cases, waiting to have cataract surgery won't harm your eye, so you have time to consider your options. If your vision is still quite good, you may not need cataract surgery for many years, if ever.

Cataracts development can be slowed, and even prevented. Of course, it helps to start early. Smoking and excessive use of alcohol can hasten cataract development as can diabetes and certain other health problems. So no smoking and only moderate alcohol. Surprisingly, excess weight is also believed a factor in cataract development. So it helps to stay slim. Wearing sunglasses that block ultraviolet B (UVB) rays can also help. And you should regularly eat a healthy diet with ample antioxidant-rich fruits and vegetables, especially yellow and dark green vegetables such as spinach and kale.

A friend who was diagnosed with macular degeneration of her eyes some 20 years ago was told by her ophthalmologist to eat spinach four times a week. This she has faithfully done. That fresh spinach sautéed in olive oil with a little minced garlic and a squeeze of lemon juice at serving has not reversed her macular degeneration, but it has halted the disease's progress.

Lutein and zeaxanthin supplements are sometimes recommended as helping prevent macular degeneration and cataracts, but there does not seem to be strong scientific evidence to support their effectiveness— especially for people who otherwise are eating a nutritionally adequate diet.

The fruit bilberry long believed beneficial for vision is rarely available in markets. Additionally, supplements containing bilberry are pricey.

Since no scientifically measurable benefit to eyes has been found, there is little justification for the expense.

The skin around the eye is particularly vulnerable to sun damage. To prevent skin cancers developing in this area, it is very important to be diligent about sunscreen and to wear sunglasses with both UVA and UVB filters. Removal of skin cancers around the eye can be disfiguring. Corrective surgery is not always successful.

Several years ago when I wrote on the *Chic & Slim* website about a family friend disfigured by skin cancer removal in the area immediately below the eye, I received an email from a woman also disfigured by such surgery. She wrote that her first corrective surgery was unsuccessful. Finally, after a period of enduring her disfigured appearance, she located a cosmetic surgeon skilled in eye-area restoration in Las Vegas and flew there for surgery. Happily this second surgery was successful.

For many of us, our eyes have been one of our most attractive features since we smiled up out of our little bassinets. With adequate attention and protection, our eyes can remain functional and attractive our entire lives.

Hands

THE MOST MEMORABLE HANDS of my childhood—surely my entire life—were those of my grandmother's friend Jeanetta. As a young woman of some beauty and equal shrewdness, Jeanetta (née Jeanie) had begun a successful career of marrying wealthy Oklahoma oil men. The exact husband count was unclear, but my grandmother who had known Jeanetta since they were young unmarried women, put the current husband, a kind, generous, charming man some years younger than Jeanetta, at number six.

Some former husbands had died, some Jeanetta had divorced, but from all the marriages she had beautiful sets of diamond wedding and engagement rings. And she wore all her rings from all her marriages every day.

Every finger on both hands wore large, sparkling diamonds. These husbands had also given her bracelets. Her wrists were roped in diamond bracelets. The brilliance from all those diamonds was almost blinding.

But her hands! By the time I knew Jeanetta, she almost 80. Her fat hands were crêpey and gnarled and covered in large dark age spots. The contrast between those ugly hands and all that beautiful jewelry fascinated me. Certainly it was Jeanetta's hands that made me a lifelong observer of hands.

So when I encountered chic French women I became immediately aware of how carefully they cared for their hands: the regular use of high quality creams— usually high in natural ingredients—how they avoided colored nail polish on fingernails, but always kept their nails perfectly manicured and buffed. If any polish was used, it was invariably clear. Not to care for one's hands was considered by chic French women as slovenly. The devoted hand care only increased in certain age.

Being such a careful observer of hands, in recent years it has pained me to see certain age women who have devoted much time and money to successfully erase signs of age on their faces, but ignored their hands that pinpoint their real age.

Today dermatologists are telling us that one major determining cause of age spots on hands is the amount of sun exposure we got when we were children and young adults. So long ago! Besides, when many of us were children we were told we needed lots of sunshine: Vitamin D for healthy bones. Sunlight was prescribed for teenage acne (my dermatologist prescribed additionally using a sunlamp when weather did not permit outdoor tanning). Many of us were certain age before medical science decided we needed sunscreen to prevent skin cancer and signs of aging. Very little of that advice on sunscreen pointed out that we needed sunscreen on our hands as well.

Of course sunscreen will only help prevent one sign of hand aging, the dark pigment spots. As we reach certain age, the fat layer on our hands begins to disappear, skin becomes wrinkly, and we (and everyone else) can see the veins, tendons and bones. Our hands start looking OLD.

When my hands began to show signs of age, I extended my anti-aging face product routine. Easy, after you put the anti-aging product on your face, rub some into the backs of your hands before you put the cap back on the bottle or tube.

The safety of using hydroquinone is debated. But there are other products designed to counter age spots for those of us who are wary. And

I have read that there are countries in the world where hydroquinone's sale is prohibited.

For daytime, that hyaluronic acid serum that I use to plump up my face gives a little volume to the tops of my hands and fingers. This, along with the liberal use of moisturizing hand creams (kept all over the house: in my office, kitchen, bathroom, beside my bed, in my handbag, in the car pocket) help counter the drying effects of hand washing and use of anti-bacterial hand gels—and the wear and tear of daily life. This hand routine does make a difference. As I can see any time there is an interruption to my upkeep program for a while.

Paraffin treatments have been around for decades as a means of softening and beautifying hands and feet—and offering pain relief to arthritic hands and feet. When I was having some laser work done on my facial hair several years ago, the technician treated me to a complimentary paraffin hand treatment with a machine the center had recently acquired. Unfortunately, the wax had not had time to cool down from the "melting" temperature to the cooler one for treatment. Though it did not blister my hand, for several days, my right hand, the first to go into the wax, was red and sore. If you have a salon paraffin treatment for your hands or feet, or acquire one of the home appliances, make sure that the wax is sufficiently cool before you plunge in your fingers or toes.

Sunscreens, creams, and exfoliation can only do so much. Particularly women who have had "medical editing" on their faces are now in the market for some of the treatments for hands to even up the results. The cosmetic medical profession is developing procedures to accommodate them. Proliferation of anti-aging treatment for hands is the big change for hands that I note from the time I wrote the first edition of *Chic & Slim Toujours*.

Hand anti-aging treatments are sometimes labeled a "hand lift." But instead of cutting and suturing, the procedure of many clinical dermatologists and cosmetic surgeons is to inject a filler such as Radiesse or Juvédern to plump up the skin. Then, a pulsed light treatment or some form of laser resurfacing to remove the age spots and encourage the production of collagen. Some physicians believe that the patient's own fat will be better accepted by the body. Instead of synthetic fillers, they will extract fat from a thigh (or other place of excess fat) and inject it into the hand.

For bulging veins, sclerotherapy, injecting a solution directly into the vein, is often the treatment of preference. Another technique is avulsions of hand veins in which veins are removed from the hands. I described this procedure in detail in that first edition of *Chic & Slim Toujours*. But avulsions seem to have been replaced by less-invasive techniques as those I have described above.

A "hand lift" is good for one to two years. But it is necessary to keep up with the sunscreen to prevent the immediate return of the age spots. The most popular anti-aging treatment for face Botox is not a choice for treating hands because it prevents mobility. But Botox is useful in treating a very annoying and to some extent debilitating condition hyperhidrosis, sweaty hands and feet.

Two of my schoolmates, one in my class, the other a few years older, suffered from this condition. The older sat next to me in a college class. Her condition was so severe that for taking notes or writing test answers, she had to keep a small terry wash cloth folded under her hand to keep the moisture from soaking the paper.

Botox injections in the hand to treat hyperhidrosis range from mildly to very painful depending on the techniques of the physician (usually a cosmetic surgeon or dermatologist) administering the Botox. Results kick in two to four weeks and will last about six months. Of course, like Botox for anti-aging, treatments for hyperhidrosis are pricey.

If you are seeking something less painful and more economical than $3000 anti-aging hand treatments with fillers, lasers and such, Karl Lagerfeld offers us a hand solution as he does for eyes. The fashion designer and creative director of Chanel now in his mid-80s is known for always wearing fingerless gloves.

Because I have a problem with my hands easily becoming numb at the slightest contact with cold (Raynaud's is not fatal, but it is often inconvenient) and more recently because of an injury to my left thumb that has resulted in arthritis there, in cold weather I wear fingerless compression gloves. Not only do these gloves combat my discomforts from Raynaud's and arthritis, but they also keep any signs of aging completely out of sight.

Well-ventilated fingerless gloves are comfortable in warm weather. You can coordinate fingerless gloves into your chic style as the designer Karl Lagerfeld does.

A CONSCIOUS GRIP

"Lose one's grip." All my life I had heard this phrase as an expression of an emotional state. That the situation had become so stressful and overwhelming that one was no longer in control of the situation—or of one's mental processes. I had no idea the phrase had its origin in the physical. Then, not long after my 70th birthday, I began to drop things.

I would be carrying a dish of catfood and it would slip from my fingers. The phrase "lose one's grip" came to mind. I did some research.

The condition, doctors tell us, is common among older people and has to do with the normal muscle and nerve changes that occur with aging. The good news is that the solution is simple and cost-free.

Previously I could carry something in my hands and my mind could be on other matters: what I was going to prepare for dinner, or the article I wanted to write for the *Chic & Slim* website. But now it was necessary to become mindful.

If I was carrying a dish of catfood to the feeding mat, I had to consciously think: I am carrying a dish of catfood, and I must keep my fingers firmly on the dish. Simple, but effective.

A conscious grip is useful when you have in your hand a dish of catfood that is replaceable. A conscious grip is absolutely essential if you have in your hand great-grandmother's antique vase that is not replaceable.

BEAUTIFULLY AGING HANDS

By the time most of us reach certain age, we will not have, as my grandmother's friend Jeanetta did, accumulated diamonds from six husbands. And wear them all every day.

But we will surely have lovely rings and bracelets we enjoy wearing and that add chic touches to our outfits. We should care for our hands so that they look as lovely as the pretty accessories with which we decorate our wrists and fingers.

Boundaries

WITHHOLDING INFORMATION ABOUT oneself has long been a successful method French women employ to set protective boundaries. The less people know about your personal affairs the better you can avoid criticism and discussions of painful subjects. The better you can avoid being the subject of gossip that could complicate your life. In the long run, the less people know about your life, the better protected you are from unhappiness and stress—and plain old annoyance.

But though this reticence about personal matters has its advantages for French women, it perhaps has contributed to the lack of boundaries to protect them from sexual harassment. In any case, French women have long been expected to deal with sexual harassment on their own. In the 16th century, Marguerite de Navarre, sister of the French Renaissance king François I, in addition to being queen of Navarre, a small kingdom in what is today southwest France, was one of the most important writers of Renaissance France. In her classic collection of short stories, the *Heptameron*, in one story, thought to be autobiographical, she tells of a young princess who has spurned the attentions of a young man at the Court. When he attempts to slip into her room at night and take her by force, she and her maid are waiting for him. Together they beat him so badly that he leaves the Court rather than explain how he came to be so badly bruised.

But in the past six years three events have prompted major changes in how sexual harassment is viewed in France.

Long after attitudes evolved in the USA, French culture still protected the private information about public figures—even in matters of sexual misconduct. Then, in May 2011, an incident in a New York hotel set change in motion. Dominique Strauss-Kahn, a former French Minister of Economy and Finance, and, at that time, director of the International Monetary Fund, was charged with a sexual attack on a hotel maid and hauled off to a New York jail.

The uproar this incident caused in France was no doubt fueled by the fact that DSK, as he was known, was likely to be the Socialist candidate in the upcoming French presidential elections—and likely the next president of France. That the maid was an immigrant to the USA from a former French colony in West Africa probably earned her extra sympathy.

In France, discussion and analysis in the media and on social media about "the DSK Affair" raged for months. Women demonstrated against sexual harassment. In France, men's inappropriate behavior began no longer to be seen as "naughtiness." Rather it was a problem for which women, especially younger French women, were demanding a remedy.

A second major event in the French attitude change toward the long-tolerated sexual predatoriness of politicians came five years later in 2016. Twelve women came forward with charges of sexual harassment against Denis Baupin, then vice-president of the National Assembly, France's lower house of Parliament. The prominent women had such credibility in their charges of inappropriate comments, fondling, and sexually explicit text messages—and the French attitude on sexual harassment had so evolved—that M. Baupin was forced to resign his position immediately.

By the time a third event occurred, the Macron administration had established a cabinet position, a Secretary of State in Charge of Equality Between Women and Men. This was no fox-in-the-hen-house appointment. The new minister was a 34-year-old woman Marlène

Schiappa that *Le Monde* described as *une blogueuse militante aux droits des femmes*, a militant blogger for the rights of women.

This third event that prompted demands for even more action against sexual harassment—by anyone toward anyone not just prominent politicians against women—like the first event, occurred in the USA.

When the sexual harassment charges against Hollywood mogul Harvey Weinstein became the most prominent topic in media and social media in the USA and punitive actions began against him, again in France it prompted increased calls for action. Demands for corrective legislation earned promises of new laws. A journalist Sandra Muller launched a Twitter hashtag *#BalanceTonPorc*, Expose Your Pig. Tens of thousands of Frenchwomen responded with their accounts of their own sexual harassment and abuse. Some, like Sandra Muller, named names.

French president Emmanuel Macron set in motion an action to strip Harvey Weinstein of his French Legion of Honor, France's highest honor, that he had been previously given for promoting foreign films. The French first lady Brigitte Macron spoke on television congratulating the women who were willing to endure their own discomfort to relate their experiences with sexual harassment and abuse.

Feminist and *New York Times* op-ed writer Lindy West wrote in the *Times* that even though it may be impossible to get legal justice for what she calls "our cultural malfunction: the smothering, delusional, galactic entitlement of powerful men," she insists that speaking out can destroy the reputations of sexual predators that silence protects.

Lindy West wrote: "We [women] don't have the justice system on our side; we don't have institutional power; we don't have millions of dollars or the presidency; but we have our stories, and we're going to keep telling them."

Speak! It is the same call that French actress Isabelle Adjani made to women of all countries and in all professions in her op-ed in *Le Journal de Dimanche* in reaction to the Harvey Weinstein exposures.

But, then, not surprisingly since this was France, a backlash occurred. In early 2018, no less than 100 prominent women, most notably the actress Catherine Deneuve, signed a letter of protest that the campaign against sexual harassment was going too far. They claimed it was threatening to upset the exceptionally good relationship between French men and women—and that it was causing French women to see themselves as victims.

Furthermore, the letter signers thought that French feminists were becoming too much like American feminists. The letter argued that French women had long been able to handle sexual harassment, and they could continue to do so.

The debate goes on.

Withholding information about a painful childhood or the amount they spent on their new winter coat gives French women a protective boundary against criticism, painful discussions, and gossip. But speaking out about inappropriate behavior is a powerful way they are attempting to build a protective boundary that those inclined to sexual harassment will be more hesitant to cross. With some legal protections, unlike the Renaissance princess Marguerite de Navarre, they will not have to hide in the dark and beat their attacker black and blue.

Aging Beautifully

LOVELY STRAIGHT POSTURE, moving smoothly like a dancer, a relaxed and smiling face, these say youth. But a stooped back, slow halting steps, and a face grimacing with pained effort, these say age. We want to avoid those signs of age. We want to age beautifully so that we look and feel young no matter how many birthdays we have celebrated.

The good news is that medical science now knows that much previously believed inevitable about aging just isn't so. Many of the bodily changes accompanying aging can be prevented, or at least slowed to the point they don't cause us too much inconvenience. Also aging is perhaps only about 30 percent genetically determined. What principally determines how quickly or slowly you age are lifestyle choices.

Lauren Kessler, author of *Counterclockwise: My Year of Hypnosis, Hormones, Dark Chocolate, and Other Adventures in the World of Anti-Aging* wrote in *Prevention* that in the Baltimore Longitudinal Study of Aging, that tracked 3,000 people from their 20s to their 90s, found not only that people age at vastly different rates, but that the older you are, the more irrelevant your birth date is to your true biological age.

Lifestyle choices greatly determine how much your biological age differs from your chronological age. You might, like the French Renaissance beauty Diane de Poitiers, be 60 but look 30, as the 16th century chronicler of women Brantôme reported.

Study after study to determine the best way to prevent the bodily changes that come aging find the solution is exercise. But most of us want an exercise that does not require three hours on horseback each morning, as Diane de Poitiers' did. We certainly want exercise that is reasonably safe. At age 64 Diane had a fall while riding horseback, with injuries so severe she never recovered. She died two years later.

We want certain age exercise that tones us and gives us strength and flexibility and the glow of health—not exercise that creates an injury that leaves us unable to exercise at all.

Exercise can solve common certain age problems. But finding the right exercise for our specific certain age problem is not always easy.

In early 2015, when I was then 71, I discovered I had a serious problem with my posture. Hard at work on another *Chic & Slim* book, I was spending long hours at the computer. The only exercise I was doing was regular sessions on the treadmill and taking brisk walks when weather permitted. In winter my old house is cold. My usual yoga and Pilates, both good for posture but requiring floor exercise, is uncomfortable. Work on the book gave me a rationale for skipping the floor exercises. By the time I realized what was going on, my standing posture had deteriorated. I was bent forward from the waist at about a 15 degree angle and my left shoulder was several inches lower than the right. Not only did I look old, I looked deformed.

I began posture correction exercises. I ordered a posture corrector, a sort of cross between a bustier and back brace. The idea behind this device seems to be that the discomfort it creates will remind you to sit and stand straight. That posture corrector is as near as I want to come to wearing a straight jacket.

I even bought wrist weights and wore only one on my right wrist in hope of leveling my shoulders. Neither the exercises, the posture corrector, nor the wrist weight made noticeable improvement in my posture.

Then, for my birthday in June, a lovely *Chic & Slim* reader Susan in Fort Lauderdale sent me Miranda Esmonde-White's book *Aging Backwards: Reverse the Aging Process and Look 10 Years Younger in 30 Minutes a Day* and the author's DVD Classical Stretch, the 30 workouts of Season 10 of Miranda Esmonde-White's public television series. Susan had inserted a pretty lavender marker at book's posture section, the first of the workouts in this anti-aging book. Her accompanying note reported that not only had these workouts improved her own posture, but given her more energy as well.

I felt confident that the Miranda Esmonde-White book and videos would provide the answer to my posture problem. Several years before Susan had sent me the Jennifer Kries Pilates workout DVD that I have written about previously in this book, one that I continue to use today. Susan knows good workout programs.

The Classic Stretch DVD posture workout uses a chair as ballet barre. I tried every chair in my house and could not find one that had the right seat height and back style to hold for support. (The DVD uses a small wicker patio chair anchored in beach sand.) So the posture exercises in the book shown with photos and step-by-step instructions done standing and on the floor were more immediately useful.

Miranda Esmonde-White's program, originally called Classical Stretch, has now been refined into one she calls ESSENTRICS, always written in all caps. For anti-aging benefits each 20-minute workout is designed as a full body workout—whether one is working toward posture improvement, or strengthening, or healing from injury.

The 12-exercise posture workout in *Aging Backwards* book began with Ceiling Reaches. This exercise proved to be key for straightening my posture. The version of Ceiling Reaches that Miranda Esmonde-White gives in the book is slightly different from the version in the warm-up on the Classical Stretch posture video, as well as the version in a video on her *essentrics.com* website.

In *Aging Backwards* she explains the Ceiling Reaches exercise's importance:

> Unless we exercise our full range of motion, we leave ourselves open to poor posture, drooping shoulders, low-energy levels and even arthritis. The solution is simple. Pull one arm at a time toward the ceiling for a total of 32 repetitions. Alternate arms with each reach. Do this consistently for 5 minutes every day.

I prefer the version of Ceiling Reaches on the Classical Stretch posture DVD with four reaches before switching arms, each reach is a bit higher and pulled slightly further back so you feel the stretch from the bottom of your abdomen all the way up to the tips of your fingers. Warning: Don't overdo this exercise at the beginning or you can make yourself very sore. Also it might be a good idea to see the demonstration of the exercise on the ESSENTRICS website so you will do it properly.

The posture correcting exercise in *Aging Backwards* of which I became most fond was the Swan. This exercise mimics a swan stretching her wings. In the learning stage, my execution was more awkward duck than elegant swan, but I loved the stretch it gave my back.

I had been working with the DVD and book exercises several months before I had time to go back and read the 115 pages of text that explain the connection between exercise and anti-aging. And from which I learned more than I ever wanted to know about the mitochondria, ligaments and tendons in my body. But here, I also found the best advice ever about good posture in certain age.

The former ballerina now anti-aging fitness expert writing about the importance of body awareness says:

> Many people's body awareness is so poor that they can stand with poor posture *feeling* [italics mine] as though they are standing correctly. It's only when they see themselves in a mirror that they realize how bad their posture actually is.

When someone becomes accustomed to poor posture, correct posture feels uncomfortable and wrong. You will need time to reprogram your mind and strengthen your muscles to achieve good posture and feel comfortable with it.

My body felt as if I had corrected my posture. When I looked in the mirror front on, my shoulders were level, yet a side view showed my back straight but I was still leaning forward from the waist at an angle. When I actually stood straight, it felt as if I was leaning backward. I helped the reprogramming of my mind as to what true straight felt like by reminding myself to "Lean Back" which was, in fact, standing straight.

I also repositioned several full-length mirrors in my house and bought a new free-standing full-length mirror and placed it where I frequently pass. With the mirrors I could constantly monitor my posture. The price of good posture in certain age is constant vigilance.

Since the *Aging Backwards* book and Classical Stretch DVD were released, Miranda Esmonde-White has released an ESSENTRICS Posture & Pain-Relief DVD that offers "age reversing full-body workouts." The posture portion is 20 minutes in length, as is the one for pain-relief. Ten minutes of how-to are included. Indicated for beginners, the DVD posture workout includes some of the exercises in the *Aging Backwards* book, but it replaces the more difficult ones.

This posture workout is effective and created with the certain age body in mind. A well-designed program. Unfortunately, the production quality of the DVD does not equal the exercise program. The videography is poor. Often the camera is so distant, or at such an angle, that it is difficult to see exactly how the exercise is performed. Oddly, though the movements of the standing exercises are elegant and flowing, the background music is, at times, a jangly, jazzy beat at a volume that makes it difficult to understand the instructions. Miranda Esmonde-White tends to chatter asides when it would be more useful to stick to giving verbal commands for the movements. But once you get the knack of the posture exercises, you can mute the sound on the DVD and provide your own background music for the workout.

If you have not yet relocated into the more leisurely realm of retirement, or if you have demanding care responsibilities for a spouse or elderly parents, or have other duties, scheduling time for exercise may present challenges. In addition to the time to actually exercise, generally exercise requires changing into exercise clothes. You must factor changing into your exercise clothes—and back into your regular clothes—into your exercise time. This makes scheduling time for exercise even more difficult.

When I learned that a strong current fashion trend in France was toward Athleisure, I was at first dismayed. Because I learned French style beginning some half century ago, my definition of chic is somewhat formal. I certainly have difficulty imagining wearing clothing designed for sports and exercise for work, shopping or social events. On the other hand, I have difficulty imagining doing Pilates in five-inch heels and a pencil skirt. The advantage I can see is that Athleisure dressing makes the transition between regular activities and exercise easier, even at times seamless. An advantage if your exercise time is extremely limited.

The other challenge working against exercise, especially in advanced certain age, is energy. Sometimes we are simply too tired from all our other have-to activities that there is no energy left for exercise. And too often those activities that leave us exhausted do not provide the exercise our muscles and heart need for good health. Those benefits must come from well-designed exercise programs.

In hindsight, it was pure folly at age 65 to take on the remodeling of an 80-year-old house and relandscaping of a half-acre property, when both house and garden were in bad states of neglect. This was especially folly in that I was still writing books, designing and maintaining a website and running a one-woman business. And that I am doing the relandscaping, interior painting and many minor repairs myself.

From beginning the project, as each year passed, I found that even with proper nutrition, exercise and adequate rest, I was too often in a state of mental and physical exhaustion.

I love my little *Provence-sur-la-Prairie* and I am not ready to give up and move to apartment or condo where someone else takes care of the yard and much of the upkeep. But what to do about my energy problem?

One way to deal with energy problems in certain age is to stop doing things that you don't much enjoy so that you have more time and energy to do the things that you do enjoy. Of course, I am not talking about necessary health and safety activities we might not like very much. What I am talking about is to stop attending the meetings of an organization that you used to enjoy, but now just doesn't seem to interest you any more. Or not always being the one who prepares and serves the big holiday dinner that becomes more exhausting every year. Let some other family member take on the job, at least for one or two holidays a year.

Or there was the woman whose very tall husband insisted that she keep the top of the refrigerator cleaned because it annoyed him to see dust accumulate there. After 40 years of keeping the refrigerator top clean, she told him she was five-foot-two and she couldn't see the top of the refrigerator so dust there didn't bother her at all. If he wanted the refrigerator top clean, he could do it himself.

DAISIES LIST

Aging beautifully is not only about remaining healthy and attractive as the years pass. Aging beautifully is also about enjoying satisfying, fun, pleasant and rewarding experiences.

I have never liked the term "bucket list," a phrase coined for those experiences you want to have and achievements you want to accomplish before you become too old to enjoy them.

But it is only the terminology I do not like—not the idea.

Definitely one should make a list of those pleasures and achievements you wish to experience before it is too late. And take some steps toward accomplishing them.

So I propose a Daisies List

"Kick the bucket" a euphemistic term for dying has a violent imagery. And buckets, while utilitarian, usually are not chic. But daisies! Daisies are lovely. Daisies are delightful. Daisies are chic.

In English we have the phrase "pushing up daisies" referring to when we are dead and buried—or our ashes interred. A much prettier metaphor than the bucket.

The food-focused French by the way, express "pushing up daisies" as *des pissenlits par les racines*, [eating] dandelions by the roots. In the USA, *pissenlits*, dandelions are considered weeds that too many people kill with applications of toxic chemicals. The French see dandelions as one of the delicious wild salad greens that make a delightful addition to a spring *salade*.

So make your Daisies List. And enjoy aging beautifully!

Resources

NUMEROUS WEBSITES AND BOOKS provided information useful to writing this book.

Wikipedia and *Google Search*, along with *Google Images* and *Google Books* were especially helpful. *Google Translate* helped out when my rusty French was stumped. *YouTube* and *Vimeo* provided helpful videos.

Many of the chic French women of certain age discussed in this book have a *Wikipedia* page, or their own website. You can find links to these websites and *Wikipedia* pages with an Internet search using your search engine of choice. Many of the women have versions of their *Wikipedia* pages and personal websites not only in French, but other languages as well. *Wikipedia's* list of alternate languages is in the left hand navigation column. Other webpages may list the name of the language, or they may have the image of a country flag to identify the link. These are generally very small and often located in the upper right corner of the webpage.

Websites of French women's magazines were valuable in providing information for this book. With their archives of articles and images, they can provide you with a wealth of additional material about topics discussed in this *Chic & Slim Toujours 2*. Even if you do not read French, you should be able to navigate the websites with easily recognizable link labels: *Mode, Beauté, Shopping, Santé* (Health). The images alone provide useful information about clothing and hairstyles. You will recognize many product names as those with which you are familiar. Some of the embedded videos, such as those for exercise or facial massage are useful even if you do not understand the accompanying voice-over instructions.

Magazine websites I found useful were: *Madame Figaro, Femme Actuelle*, French *Elle*, French *Vogue*, French *Marie Claire*, French *Huffington Post, Gala, Point de Vue, Le Point, Paris Match, Europe1,* and *L'Express*.

France24.com, Amazon.fr, Sephora.fr, fnac.com, auFeminin.com, and *linternaute.com* websites were also helpful.

The French newspapers *Le Figaro, Le Parisien, France Soir, Libération, La Voix du Nord, L'Action Agricole Picarde, Le Courrier Picard, Le Journal de Dimanche,* and *Le Monde* provided background information. As did the Swiss daily newspaper *Le Temps*.

Several newspapers in the UK cover French topics well. I found useful information on websites of *The Guardian, Times Online, The Telegraph, The Independent, The Daily Mail, The Financial Times,* and *BBC News*. The *Daily Mail* is the best source of full-length color photos of chic women, both French and other nationalities.

The US magazines *Harpers Bazaar, Prevention, Shape, Marie Claire, Allure, Slate, Vogue* and *New York* magazine provided information.

In the USA, the best coverage of France and chic French women is *The New York Times*. Less frequently you can find articles about chic French women in *The Washington Post* and *The Los Angeles Times*. *The Huffington Post* also covers France and French culture in English as well as in their French language edition.

Websites of cosmetics companies provided information about these companies and their products. You can learn more about these on their websites, and in some cases, learn the location of a store in your area that sells their products. *Dermstore* and *Sephora* websites also provided information and user reviews about products and their best use.

Websites of beauty institutes and clinics in France and the USA provided information about spa and medical treatments. You can learn more about beauty treatments in France on the websites of the *Institut des Jambes* Rennes, *Biologique Recherche, Darphin Vendôme Institute,* and *Massage Vichy* among others.

Paris facialist Joelle Ciocco has a frequently updated blog in English as well as French with many articles about skin care.

The website *Mountain Rose Herbs* has good information and sells the ingredients for making your own beauty products from herbs and essential oils. Another excellent source of information about essential oils is Sally Wong's *Think Oily* blog.

Footwear News has frequently updated information about fashionable shoes—and celebrities who wear them.

The websites of National Institutes of Health (NIH), *Stylecaster, The Cut,* and *Yahoo News* also provide information related to subject matter in this book. I found Kathleen Hou's articles in *The Cut* particularly useful.

Various internationally known beauty specialists are generous in sharing their expertise and advice via their websites and videos both on *YouTube* and *Vimeo.* You can easily find them with web searches.

The website for Miranda Esmonde-White's exercise programs is *essentrics.com.* Exercise videos mentioned in this book: *Classical Stretch: The Complete Season 10 TV Series*, The Esmonde Technique, 2014 and *Posture & Pain Relief for Beginners,* The Esmonde Technique 2015.

Books provided useful information about chic French women's beauty treatments and other topics. These included:

Sarah Bakewell, *At The Existentialist Cafe: Freedom, Being, and Apricot Cocktails,* Chatto & Windus, 2016.

Miranda Esmonde-White, *Aging Backwards: Reverse the Aging Process and Look 10 Years Younger in 30 Minutes a Day,* Harpers, 2014.

Linda Dannenberg. *The Paris Way of Beauty.* Simon & Schuster, 1979.

A. Norman Jeffares, ed. *Yeats the European*. Rowman & Littlefield, 1989.

Princess Michael of Kent. *The Serpent and the Moon*. Touchstone, 2004.

Nicole Ronsard. *Cellulite: Those Lumps, Bumps, and Bulges You Couldn't Lose Before*. Beauty & Health Publishing Corp., 1973.

Carol Sabas. *Fashion Insiders' Guide to Paris*. Abrams, 2013

Mathilde Thomas. *The French Beauty Solution: Time Tested Secrets to Look and Feel Beautiful*. Penguin Random House, 2015
  Note: An excellent book on the French traditional approach to beauty with many practical recommendations and DIY recipes for traditional French beauty treatments.

Kathleen Wellman. *Queens and Mistresses of Renaissance France*. Yale University Press, 2013.
  Note: *Queens and Mistresses* contains much interesting information about these women, but sadly the book is not well-written, nor well-edited. Because of its high price, if you are interested in reading it, you might want to borrow it from your library or via interlibrary loan.

Charles Van Doren. *The Joy of Reading: A Passionate Guide to 189 of the World's Best Authors*. Harmony/Crown, 1985.

Christine Valmy. *Christine Valmy's Skin Care and Makeup Book*. Crown Books, 1982.

For more information related to the topics discussed in this book and information about living chic and slim *à la française*, visit the *Chic & Slim* supporting website *annebarone.com*.

Merci Beaucoup

THE MORE YEARS THAT PASS, the harder to find time and energy for all that I plan to write. Assistance is needed and greatly appreciated.

Our indefatigable *Chic & Slim* Special Correspondent Kat in London and France keeps me up-to-date with personal reports, articles, and photos on matters chic and slim—not only in France and the UK, but from other points of her travels.

Without the exercise books and DVDs Susan in Fort Lauderdale has provided me through the years, I would not feel as well, nor be as able to manage my posture so necessary for health and chic.

Susan in Hamilton ships me a wealth of books and magazines that provide information on style and decor. These help not only with chic and slim topics, but are guides for my house and garden remodeling projects here at *Provence-sur-la-Prairie*.

Ann Leslie in New York can always locate and send links to the most complete information on even the most esoteric subjects. Her expertise in art, music, food and gardening is invaluable.

Vicki in Friday Harbor continues to inspire me with examples of elegant design and send me letters and emails of encouragement that seem to arrive at most needed times.

Karen in Rosemount saved me from an embarrassing mistake about a tea in a website article and often sends useful links, most notably the link to the photos of Cotterstock Hall and its Dryden Room, my bedroom on visits to that 17th century English mansion.

Jane in Dallas sent articles to which I would otherwise not had access that alerted me to major new trends in facial care useful for the book.

Joyce in Griggs also frequently emails encouragement. For this book she provided a generous quantity of supplies that spur my creativity and facilitate the writing. She also designed the Eiffel Tower design that appears in the books and on the *Chic & Slim* website.

My son John, though recovering from illness, fortified himself with cups of hot tea to edit this book. His collections of "tea reading" arrive regularly and provide background information for the *Chic & Slim* books and website articles.

Faithful *Chic & Slim* readers far too numerous to name individually regularly send helpful links, useful information, apt comments, and much-appreciated thanks. I especially enjoy knowing how the books and website have helped them live chicer, slimmer and happier lives.

To all of you, my deepest gratitude.

Merci beaucoup!
Anne Barone

For more information
on topics covered in this book
and ordering other *Chic & Slim* books
visit the *Chic & Slim* supporting website

annebarone.com

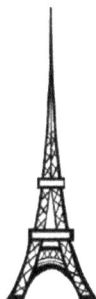

www.ingramcontent.com/pod-product-compliance
Lightning Source LLC
Chambersburg PA
CBHW072014040426
42447CB00009B/1632